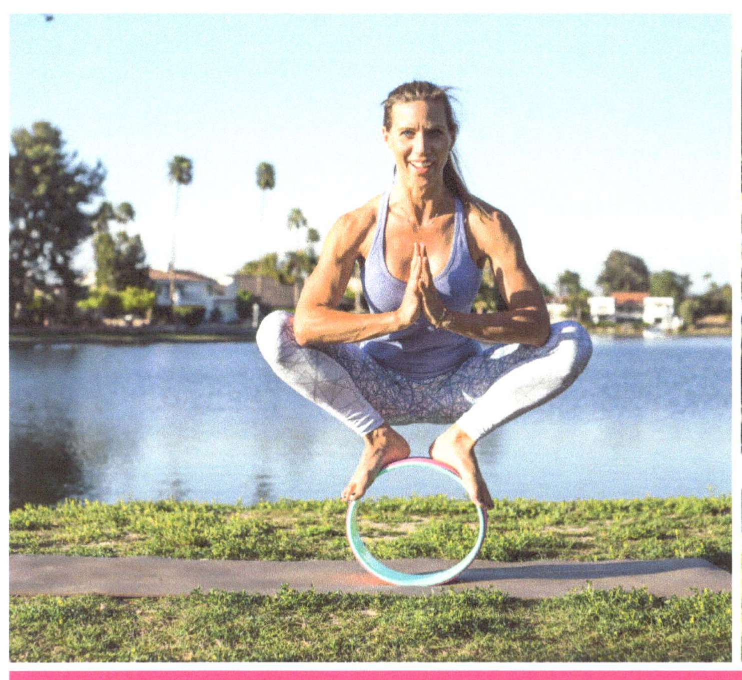
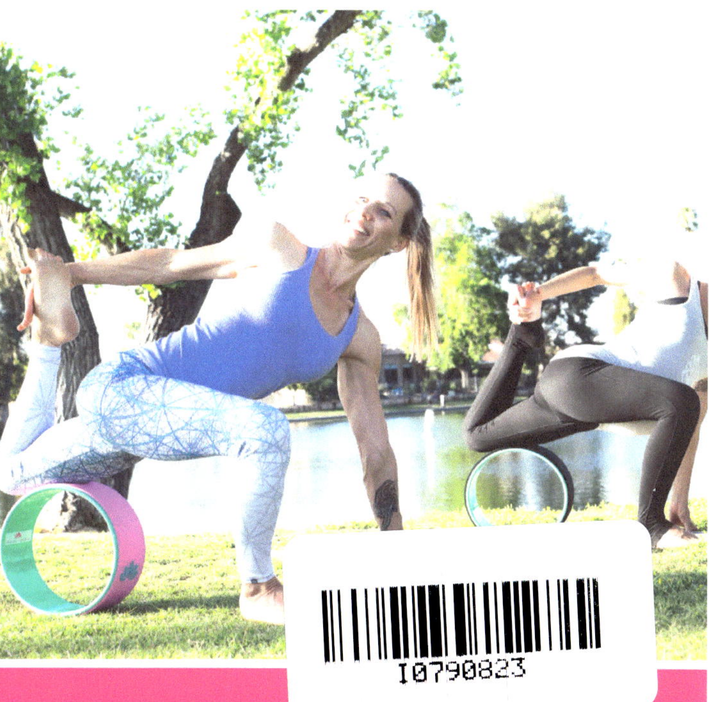

THE
SHAKTI YOGA WHEEL
98 POSTURE GUIDE

SCOTTSDALE | MUNICH

www.shaktiyogawheel.com

Revised Version 1.2.

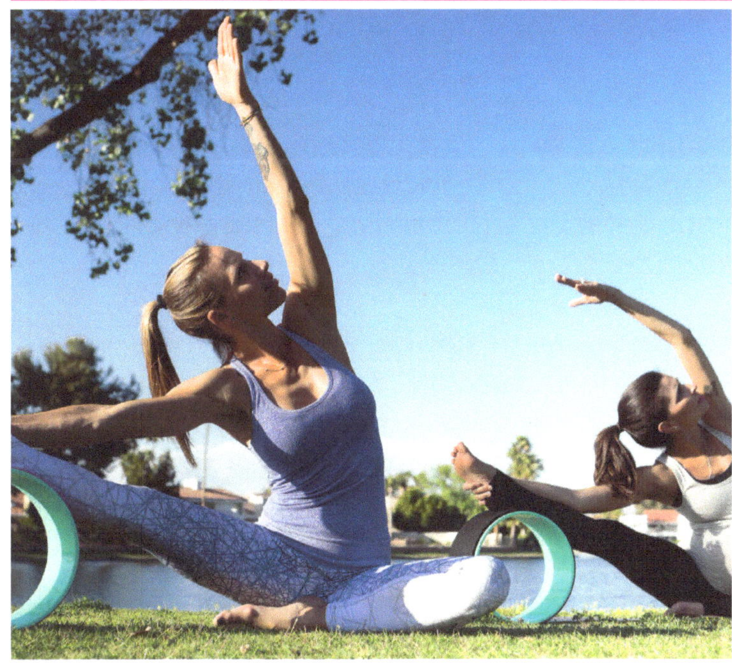
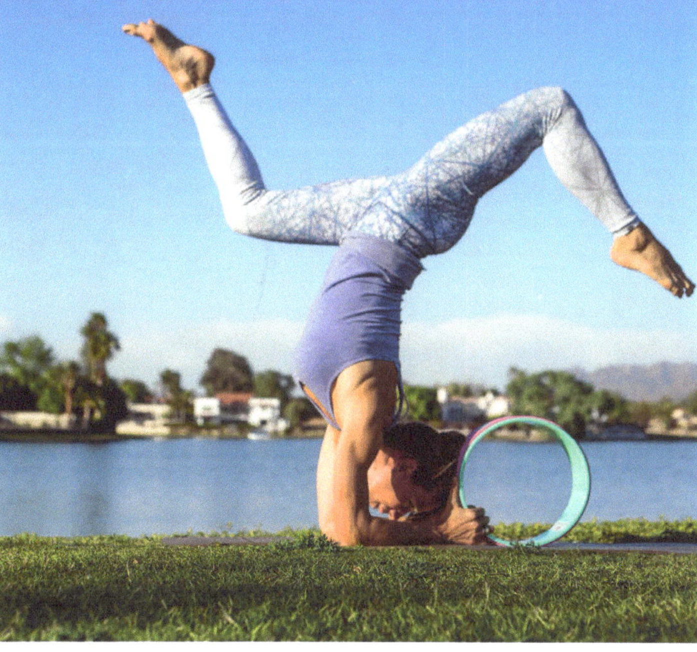

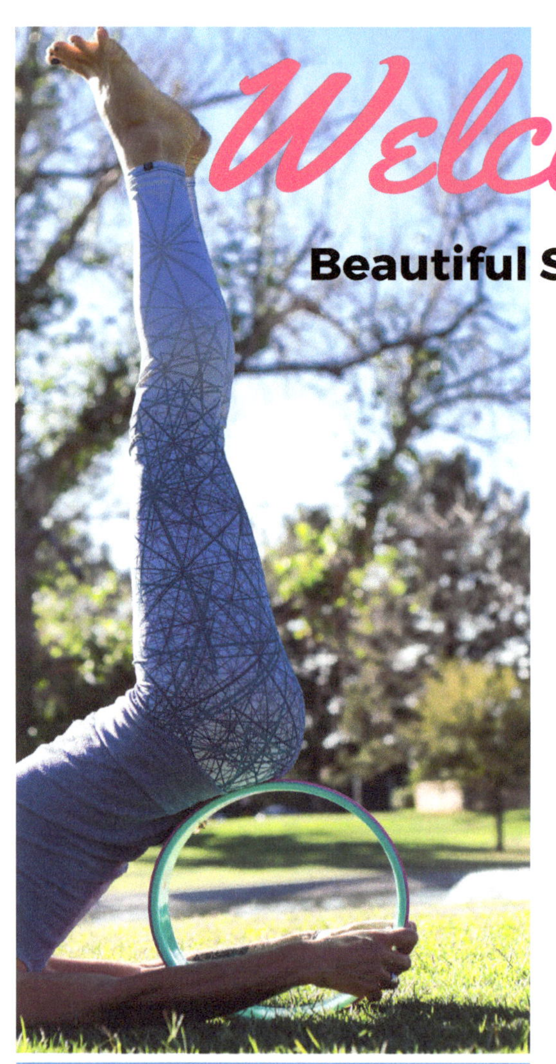

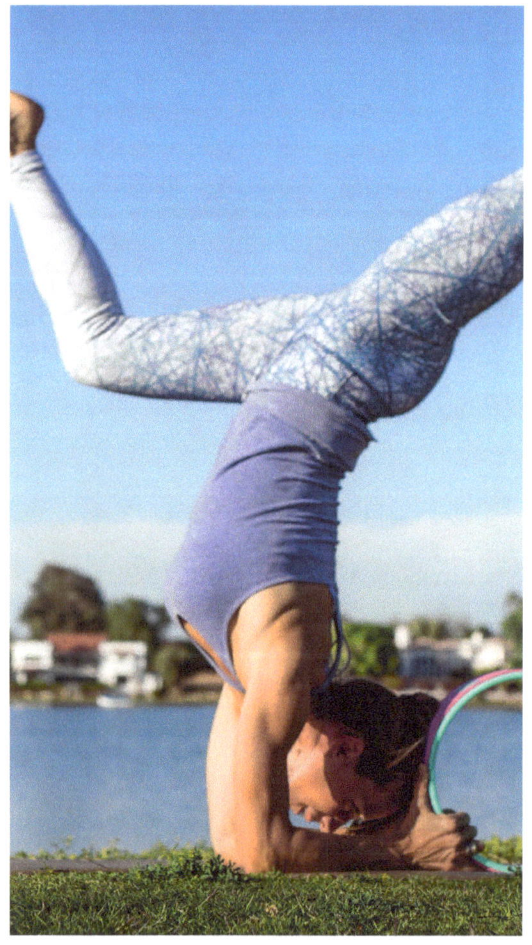

Welcome

Beautiful Souls!

We dance to a different beat. We stretch with the yogis, run to the highest peaks, travel to unexplored territories, and swim where the oceans become one.

We are delighted to share the revised Shakti Yoga Wheel™ - 98 Posture Guide with you! When we first published the guide in 2016, it was a huge success. This guide was a comprehensive photo manual for yoga practitioners who wanted to know how to incorporate the yoga wheel into their practice. As the yoga wheel practice is becoming even more popular, we decided to revise the guide by adding in-depth instructions for each pose, so that people of all levels can benefit from using The Shakti Yoga Wheel.

If you have questioned if a yoga wheel will be useful in your practice, you will be exuberantly happy to find each and every yoga wheel posture particularly described.

With this guide you will discover how the yoga wheel supports your practice, allowing you to experience a fuller expression of each pose. We are sure The Shakti Yoga Wheel™ will become an invaluable new tool for your practice.

In this Shakti Yoga Wheel – 98 Postures Guide you will find a variety of exercises, poses, and flows to help strengthen your core, increase your flexibility, improve your balance and stability, and deepen your backbends.

When practicing with this guide and your yoga wheel, you will move through familiar poses while you challenge new muscles. You will experience a well-rounded yoga class, leaving you feeling free-spirited, light-hearted, blissful, and more receptive. By the end of your practice, you will surely know how to do more than simply roll around on your wheel!

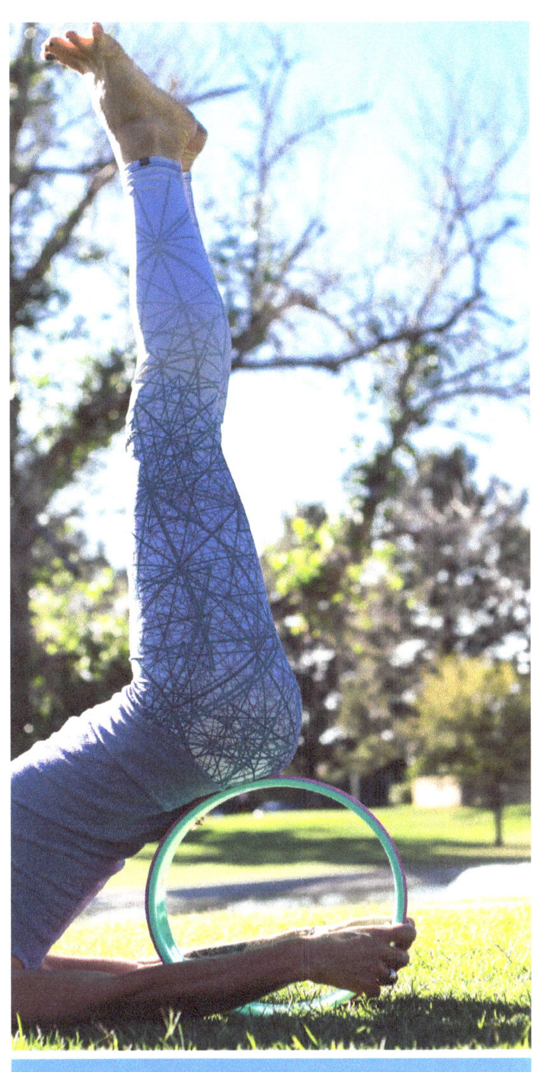

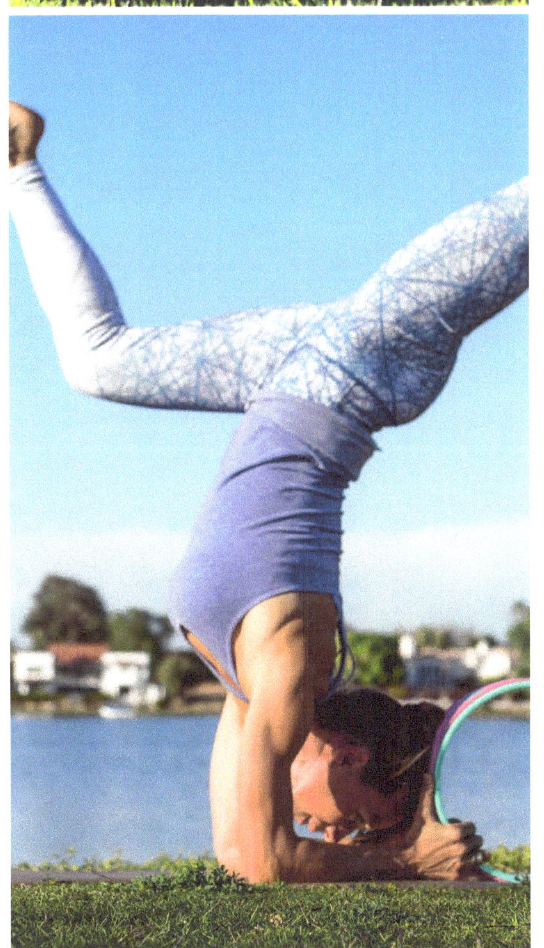

The yoga wheel is heavily inspired by the yoga pose urdva dhanurasana, (wheel pose.) Wheel pose has long been a favorite posture for opening up the chest and bringing flexibility and mobility to the spine. For most students, however, practicing deep backbends like urdva dhanurasana is very difficult and even painful. The Shakti Yoga Wheel™ will help you achieve backbends safer and with greater ease. Practicing deep backbends will open the solar plexus chakra, increasing feelings of self-worth, self-power, and self-esteem in the practitioner. We couldn't think of a better feeling, and so The Shakti Yoga Wheel™ was born.

Open your heart and grow like a lotus; this is our motto. For us, it embodies the essence of the yoga teachings, which is to embrace life with acceptance and grace, no matter the situation. Shakti Yoga™, which was founded in 2005, is not just a brand, but it is a way of living and loving fully.

Before practicing on your Shakti Yoga Wheel™

- We always recommend a warm up before starting to work with a yoga wheel
- We recommend a regular yoga practice for at least 6 months
- In some postures you will put pressure on the abdomen, so please be sure to eat about two hours before your practice begins to allow your food to digest
- Many of the postures are recommended for women in pregnancy as well. However, we advise you to talk to your doctor before beginning practice on the yoga wheel. Always avoid postures where you place the wheel on the belly.

Shine like the whole universe is yours

~Rumi~

Contents

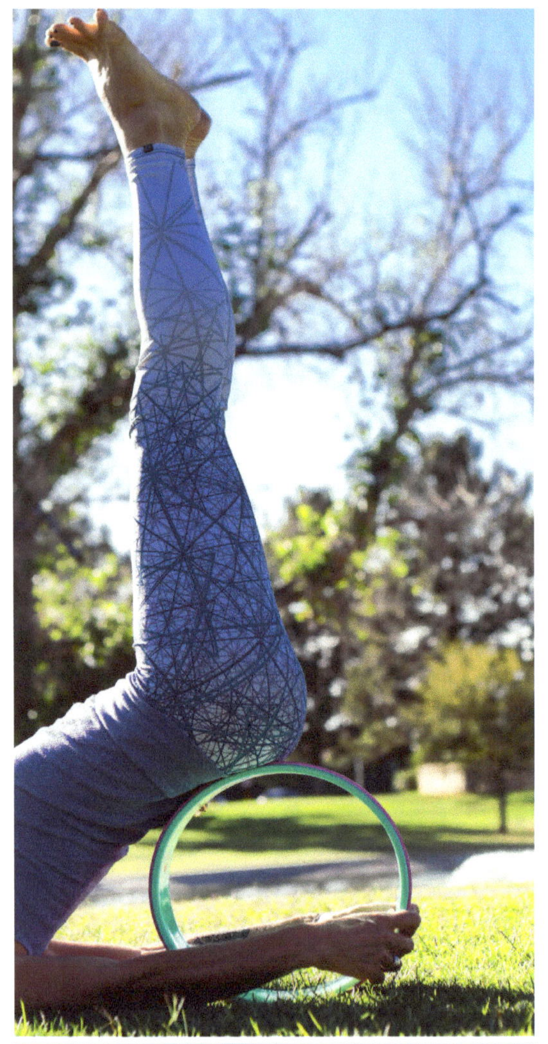

Thank You Notes & Author
Safety information

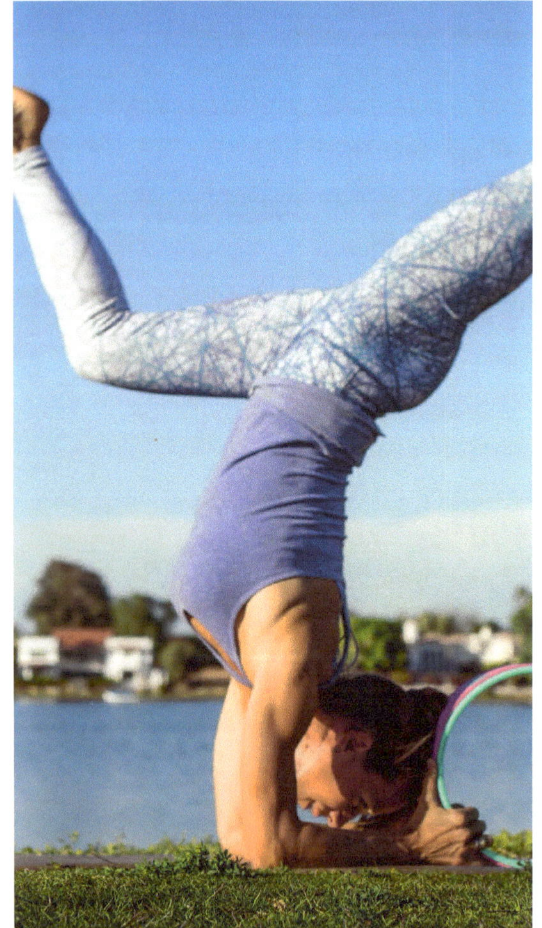

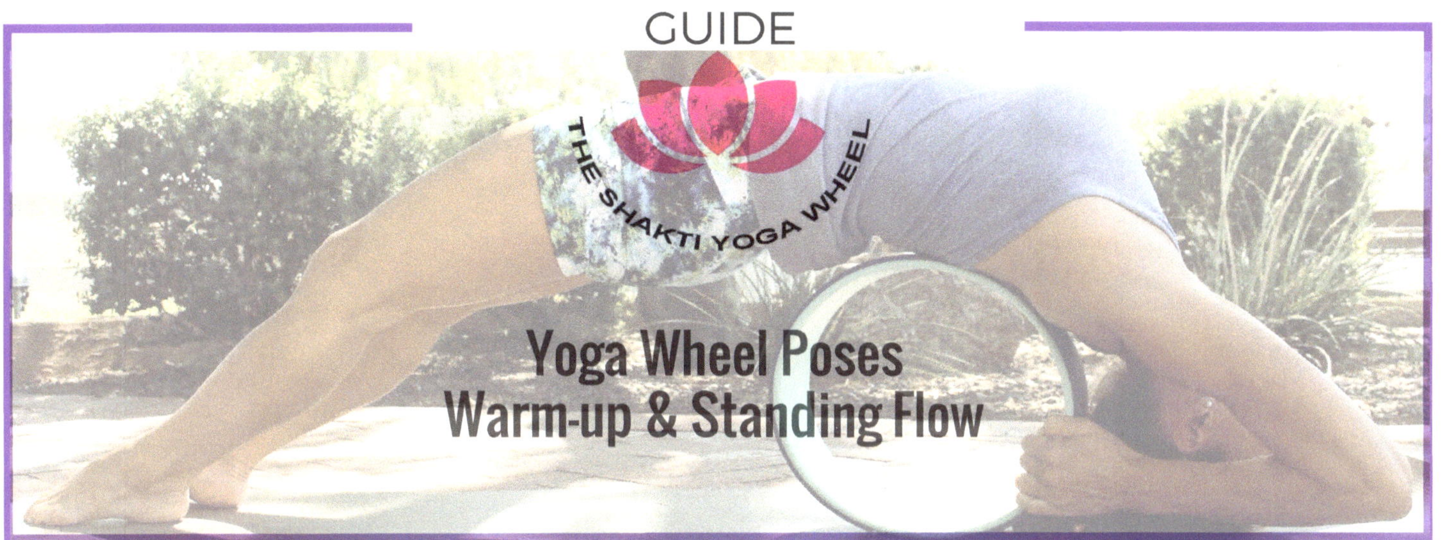

Yoga Wheel Poses
Warm-up & Standing Flow

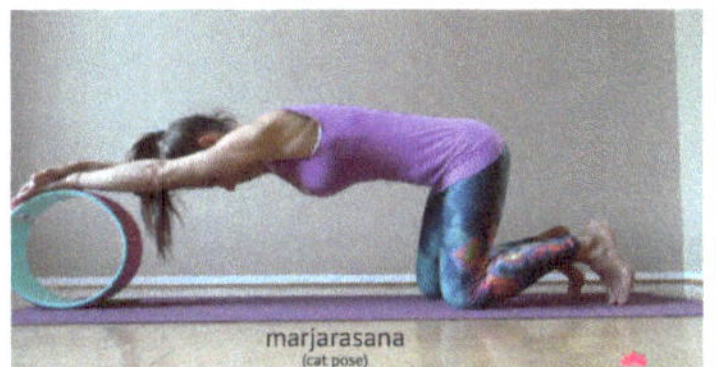

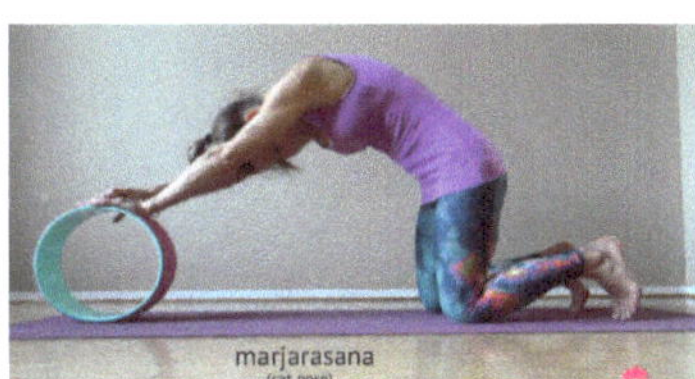

Marjarasana - (cat-cow pose)

Start on hands and knees, with your shoulders over wrists and your hips over knees. Place one hand on top of the wheel, and then place the other hand on top of the first hand. Tuck your toes and on an inhale breath, begin to roll the wheel away from you, dropping your heart and gazing forward and up. Visualize the shoulder blades and bring the outer edges of the shoulder blades in towards the spine. Keep your navel drawing back toward the spine as you stretch through the front of the body. Press into the palms to lift your inner armpits.

On an exhale breath, tuck your chin to your chest and with straight arms, roll the wheel in towards you. Draw both sides of the waistline back and press the back of your heart to the sky, expanding through the back body. This should feel much like a sit-up, where the front of the body is contracted and drawing in.

Roll the wheel in and out a few times, moving with your breath, and then switch the palms so that the other hand is on top.

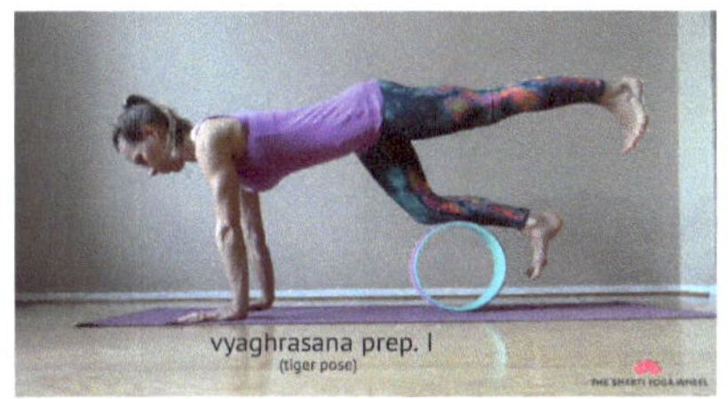

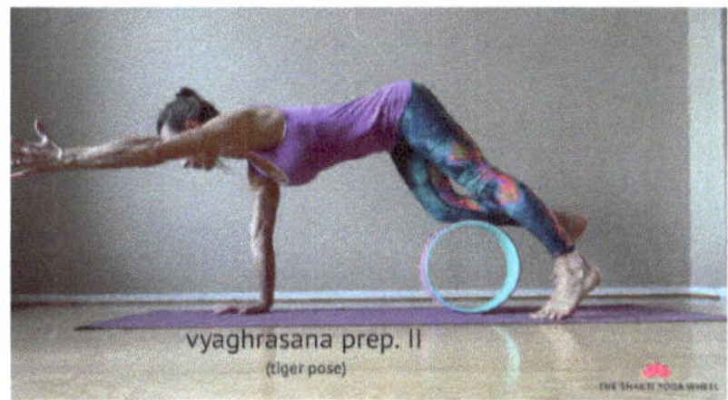

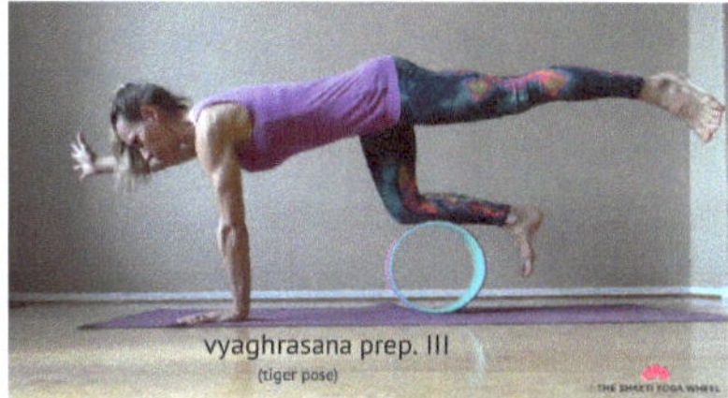

Vyaghrasana prep. I -(tiger pose)

From hands and knees, tuck the toes and press up into downward facing dog. Roll the wheel back towards your feet, lift one leg, and place that shin on top of the wheel just below the knee, at the top of the shinbone. Flex the foot of that leg strongly. Hug to the midline by firming the forearms in towards each other and engaging the inner thigh muscles. Press into your palms, draw both sides of the waistline back and see if you can lift your planted downward dog foot off of the mat.

Vyaghrasana prep. II - (tiger pose)

Keep the wheel where it is underneath the shinbone and place the lifted leg back onto the mat. This time we will try to lift the opposite arm. Engage your core and find your center as you lift the palm up off the mat and sweep the arm forward, bicep in line with the ear.

Vyaghrasana prep. III - (tiger pose)

Now we put vyaghrasana prep. I and II together and we try it with one leg lifted as well as one arm lifted. Of the leg that is on the wheel, continue to flex the toes back toward the shin. Press into your hands, draw the navel to the spine, and lift the planted downward dog foot off of the mat. Isometrically drag your palms back toward the wheel. Lift the arm that is opposite of the lifted straight leg and sweep it forward, bicep in line with the ear. *Rest in child's pose if needed before placing the wheel on the other shin and trying all three variations on the second side.*

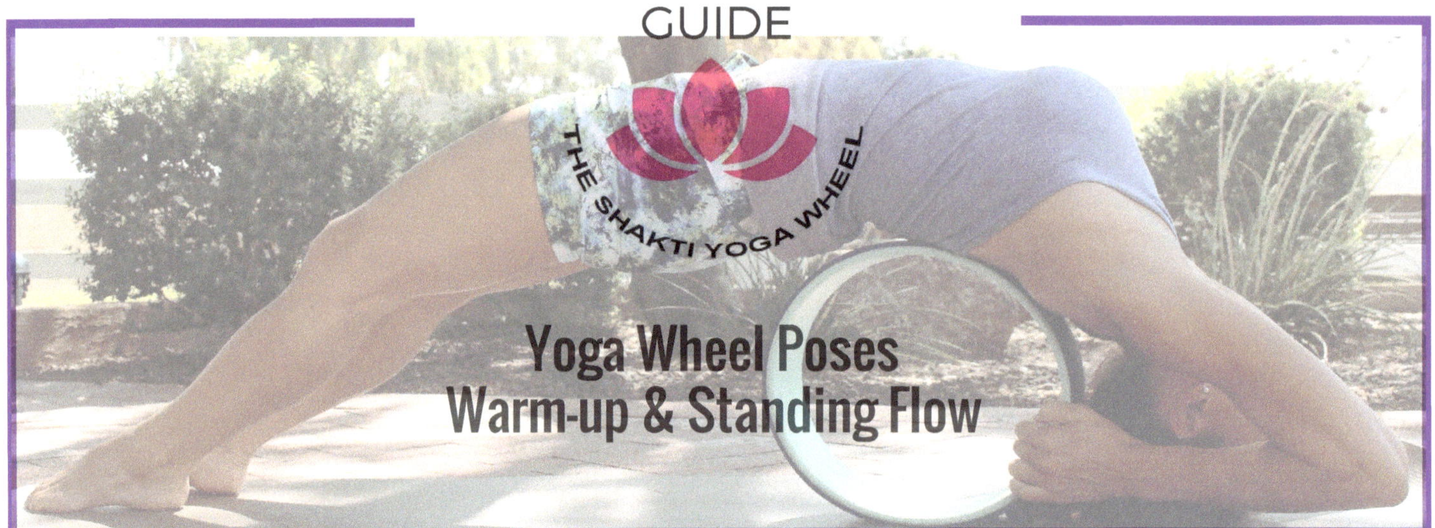

Yoga Wheel Poses
Warm-up & Standing Flow

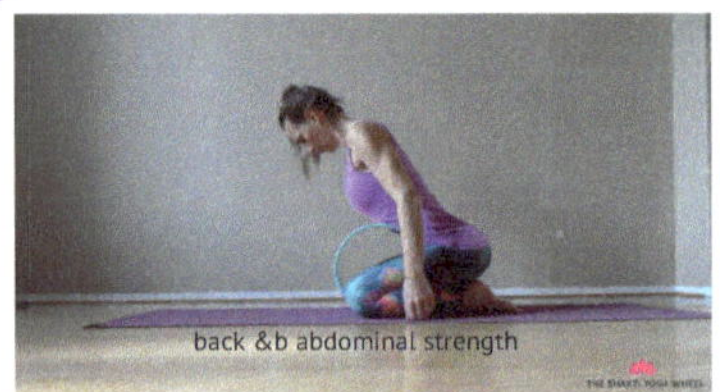
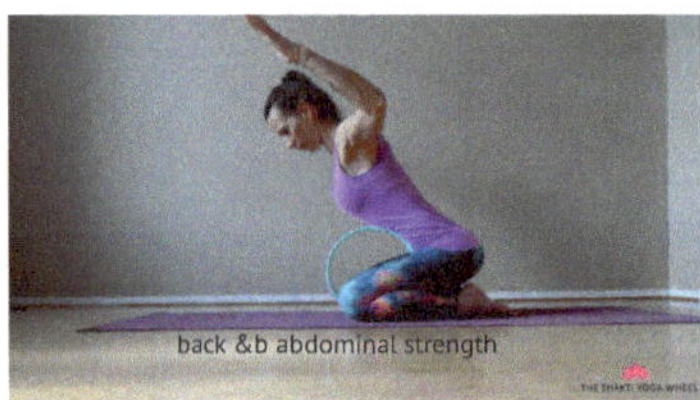
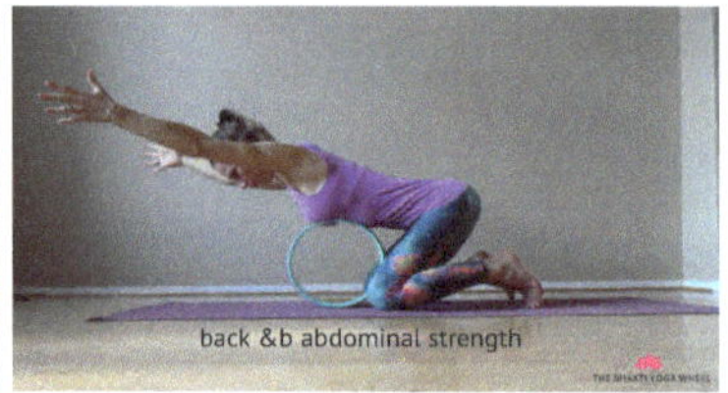

Back & abdominal strength - variation I
Come to your knees, press the tops of the feet into the mat and sit back onto your heels. Roll the wheel in between your thighs and lean forward to rest the front of your torso against the wheel. Play with the wheel and place it wherever it is most comfortable. Slightly tuck the chin to the chest, pull the sternum in and firm the outer edges of the shoulder blades in toward the spine. Pull the belly in and up. Create a curve in the low back and lengthen the spine, extending through the top of your head and out through the base of the spine.

Back & abdominal strength - variation II
Bend your elbows to 90-degrees and come to "goal post" or "cactus" arms. Squeeze the shoulder blades in and engage the muscles of the upper back. Continue to draw the sternum in, but allow the heart the shine out.

Back & abdominal strength - variation III
If everything is feeling right in your core and in your back, extend the arms out in front of you. Tuck the chin, pull the sternum back and lift the armpits. Then lengthen through the top of your head, slide the ears back and squeeze the shoulder blades in.

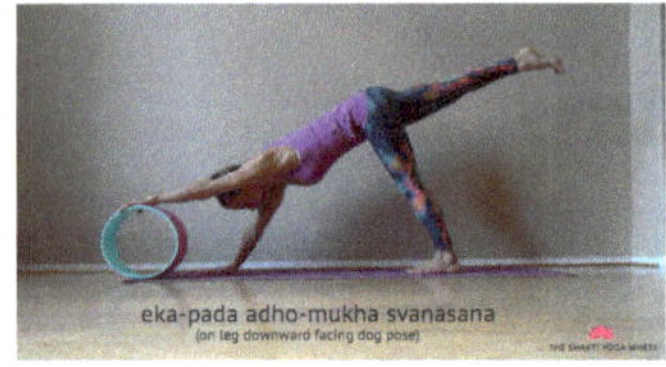
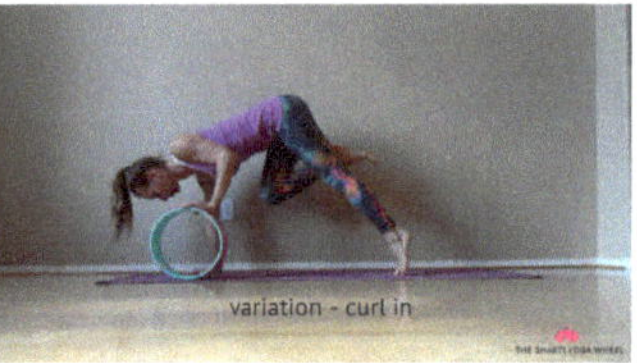
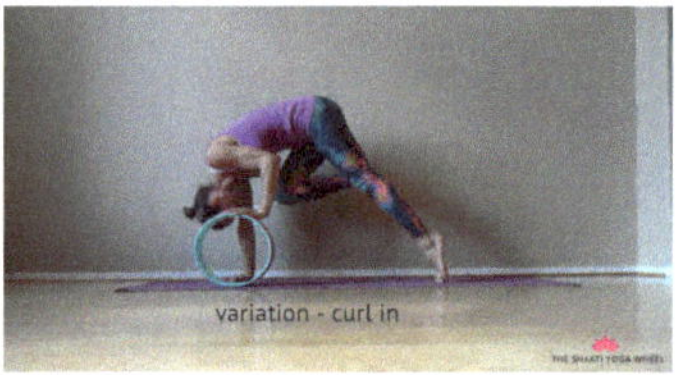
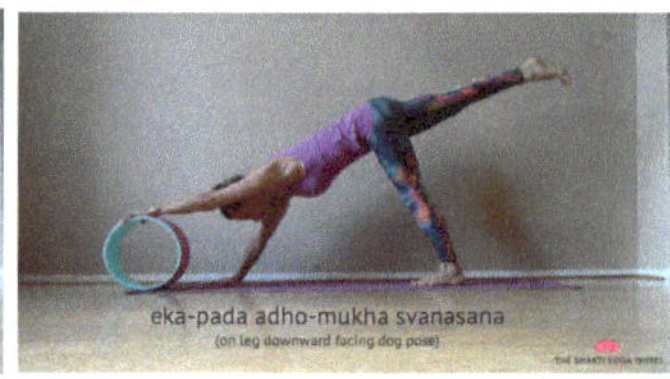

Eka-pada adho-mukha svanasana - (one leg downward facing dog pose)
Begin in downward facing dog with the wheel underneath one of your palms. Press both hands down to lift the inner armpits and to draw the waistline back. With one hand on the wheel, lift the opposite leg up to a 3-legged downward facing dog pose, keeping the hips square and level, toes pointing down to the mat.

Eka-pada adho-mukha svanasana variation - (one leg downward facing dog pose knee to chest)
From there, bend the lifted leg and bring the knee forward under your navel. Roll the wheel back towards the knee, pulling the wheel and knee closer together. Press into both palms.

Eka-pada adho-mukha svanasana variation - (one leg downward facing dog pose knee to nose)
For more challenge, tuck the chin to the chest and bring the knee all the way forward to the nose rather than to the navel. Lift both sides of your waistline back, contract the front body, and expand into the back body.

Eka-pada adho-mukha svanasana - (one leg downward facing dog pose)
After curling the knee into the wheel, inhale to roll the wheel away from you and lengthen the leg back to 3-legged downward facing dog.

Try this knee to navel or knee to nose 3 times.

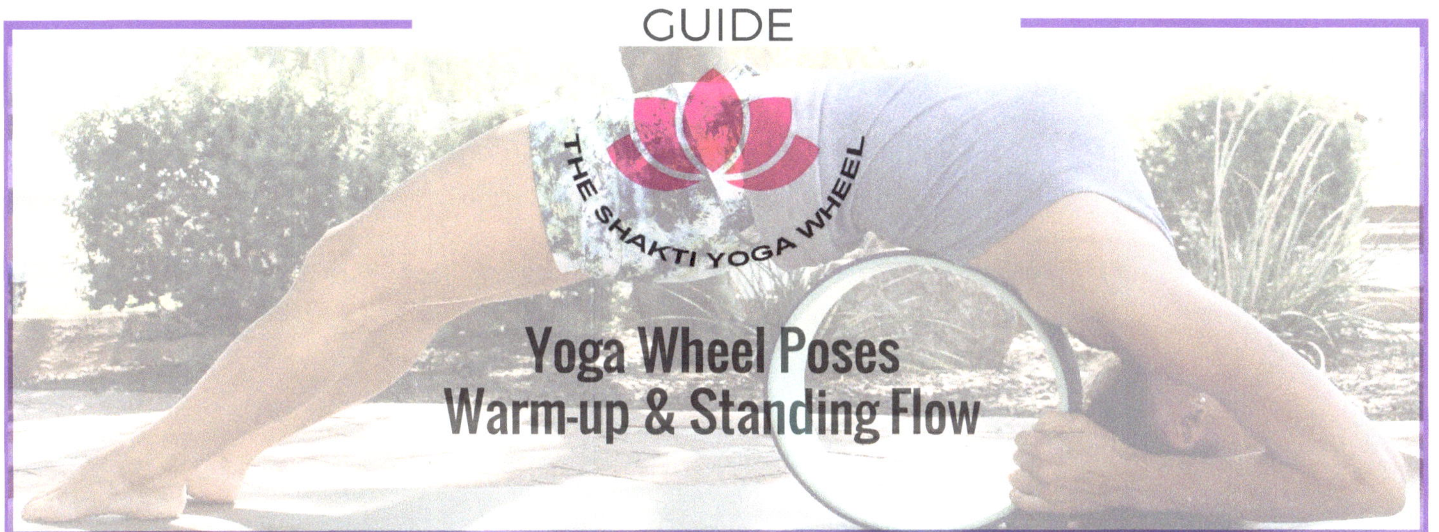

Yoga Wheel Poses
Warm-up & Standing Flow

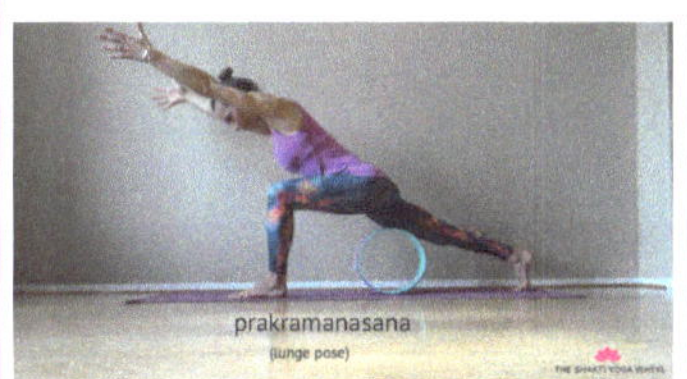

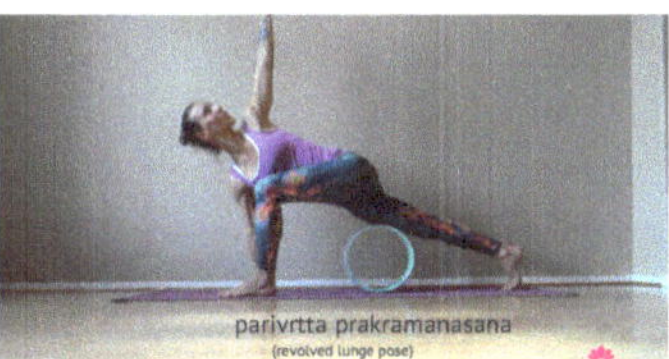

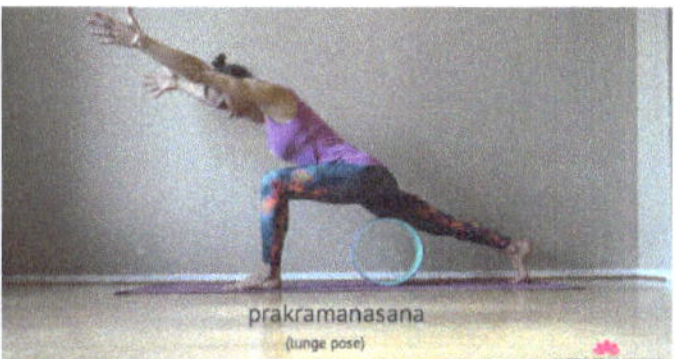

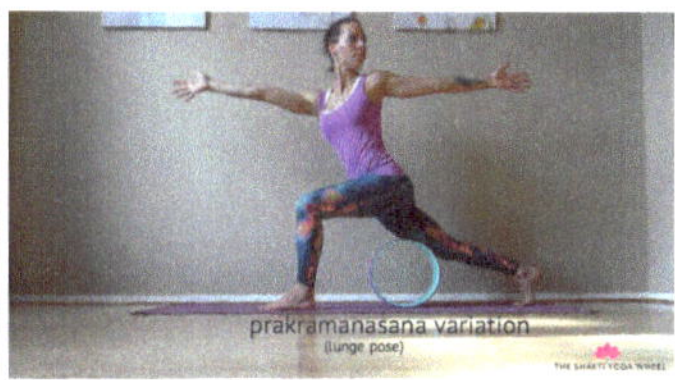

Prakramanasana variation - (lunge pose)
From 3-legged downward facing dog, hug the knee into the chest and step the foot to the front of the mat, between your thumbs. Roll the wheel to the back of the mat, placing it under the back thighbone. Place the wheel wherever it is most comfortable. Scissor the hips so that you pull the outer edge of the front hip back and allow the outer edge of the back hip to come forward. Squeeze the feet towards one another and hug the outer hips in. Feeling light on your fingertips, begin to float the arms up to a 45-degree angle. Use the wheel for stability and press the thighbone into the wheel. Pull your belly away from the front thigh.

Parivrtta prakramanasana - (revolved lunge pose)
Begin to twist your heart toward the front leg, rotating your ribs toward the inner thigh of that front leg. Place one palm down onto the mat. Your top arm can touch the front knee, the front hip, or it can extend up toward the sky. Lift your back inner thigh up and press the wheel forward.

Prakramanasana variation - (lunge pose)
Come back to the lunge with your arms extended at a 45-degree angle in front of you.

Prakramanasana variation - (lunge pose)
Firm the outer hips in, keep squeezing the feet together, and float your upper body all the way up. Open your arms to the sides, palms facing up, and twist in the same direction as before. Pull the front outer hip back and gaze to the back of the mat.

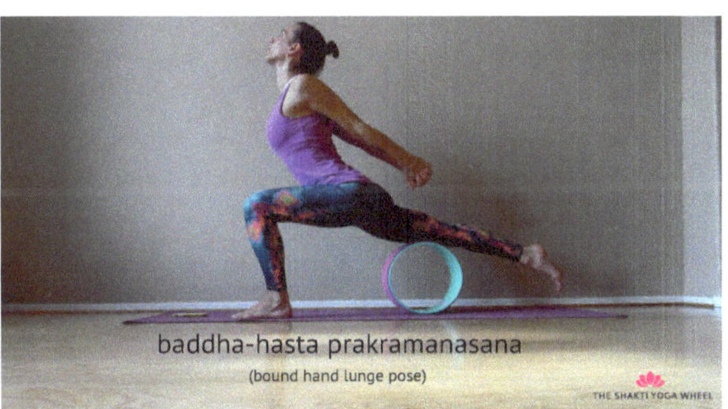

Baddha-hasta prakramansana - (bound lunge pose)
Untwist your pose and return to facing to the front of the mat. Reach your arms back behind you and interlace your fingers at your low back. Slightly tuck the chin to the chest, draw the sternum back and roll the heads of the arm bones up and back. Now glide your ears back, lift your heart, and squeeze the outer edges of the shoulder blades together. Visualize the bottom tips of the shoulder blades picking up your heart. Press the heart and the top of the front shinbone more forward as you lift the ball of the back foot off of the mat.

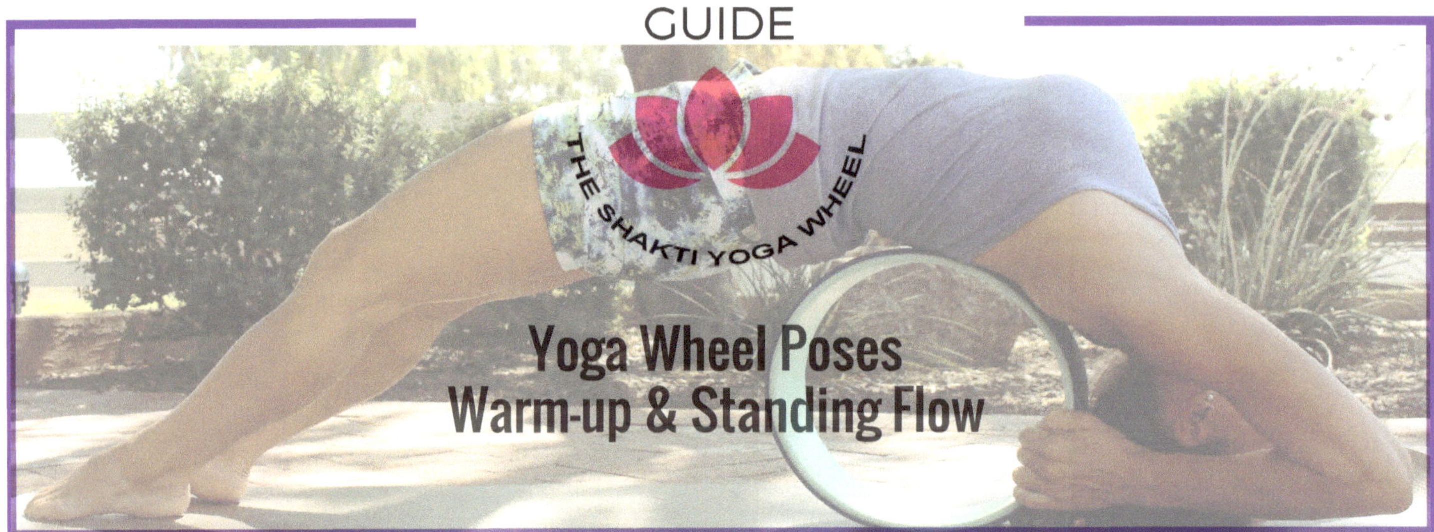

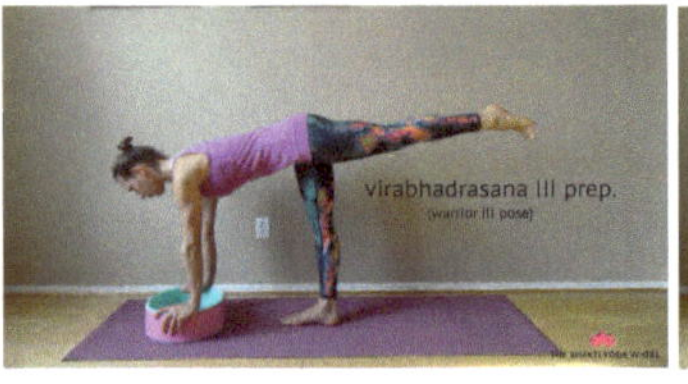

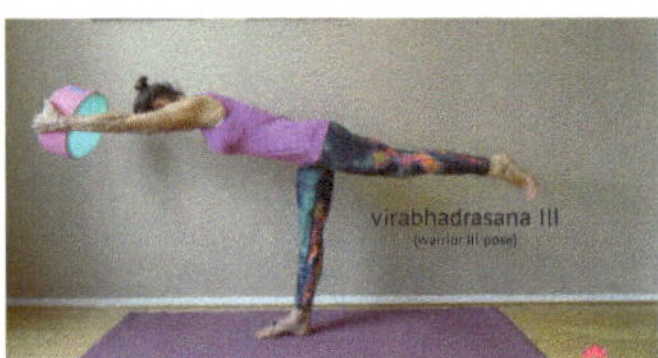

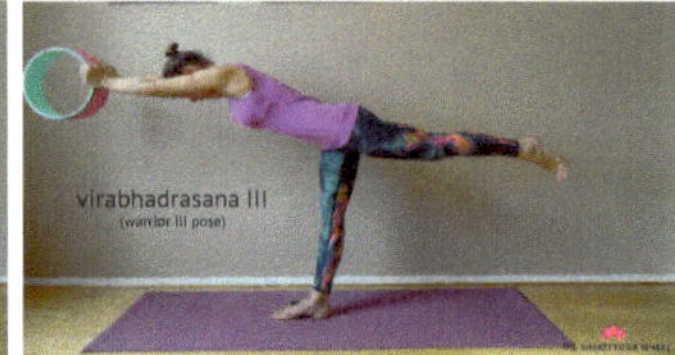

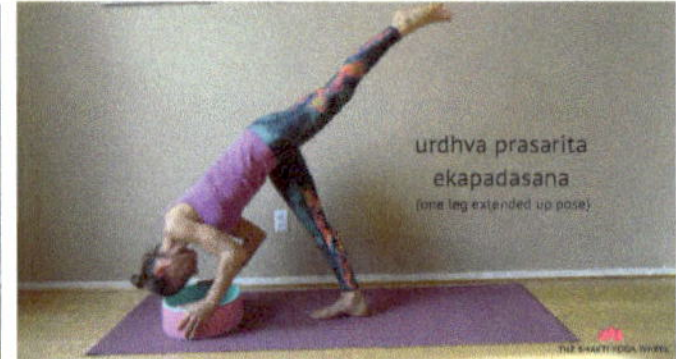

Virabhadrasana III prep. - (warrior III pose)

From bound lunge pose, release your hands to the mat. Reach back and grab the wheel and lay it on its side at the front of your mat. Press your hands into the edges of the wheel and step on the front foot, floating the back leg up to hip height. Bend your standing leg if needed to reach the wheel lying on the floor. If you are more flexible, be careful that you do not hyperextend the standing knee. Press the top of the shinbone forward to keep that knee active and engaged. Keep your hips square and level by pointing the back toes down to the mat. From the standing foot, pull energy up to the top of the thighbone. Lift the kneecap, the quadriceps, and the low belly up. Draw both sides of the waistline back. Extend out through the top of your head and the inner edge of the back foot.

Virabhadrasana III - (warrior III pose)

If you feel strong here, grab the wheel and lift it off of the mat, extending the arms and the wheel out in front of you, biceps in line with your ears. Think of making one long line of energy from the wheel to the lifted back foot. Draw the navel to the spine and root down into the standing foot.

Virabhadrasana III variation - (warrior III pose)

This variation has you holding the wheel in a narrow grasp, rather than the wider one as in the previous photo. Squeeze the shoulder blades in and pull the waistline back.

Urdhva prasarita ekapadasana - (standing splits pose)

Bring the wheel back to the mat and lie it down on its side. Begin to hinge at the hips as you kick the lifted leg higher. You are like a see-saw here; as one side drops down, the opposite side lifts up. With the back toes pointing down to the mat, lift the inner thigh up as you drop the outer thigh down. Fold as deeply as you like, bending your elbows and lowering the head to the wheel.

Don't forget the second side!

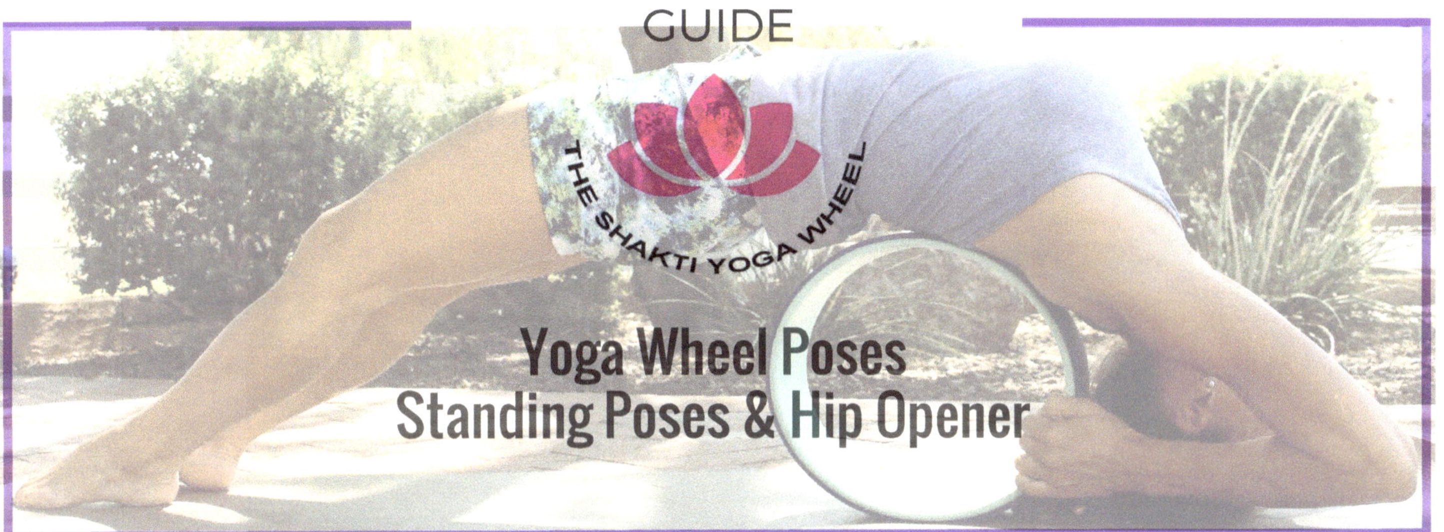

Yoga Wheel Poses
Standing Poses & Hip Opener

Begin in tadasana (mountain pose) for all of the standing poses. These one legged, standing poses require a solid, centered foundation. Firm your muscles to the midline of your body to find that center. From the inner edges of the feet draw energy up the legs to the low belly, engaging the calf, knee and upper thigh muscles along the way. Lift the low belly up and draw the navel back to the spine. Narrow the front ribs and slide them down to feel a strong connection to your core.

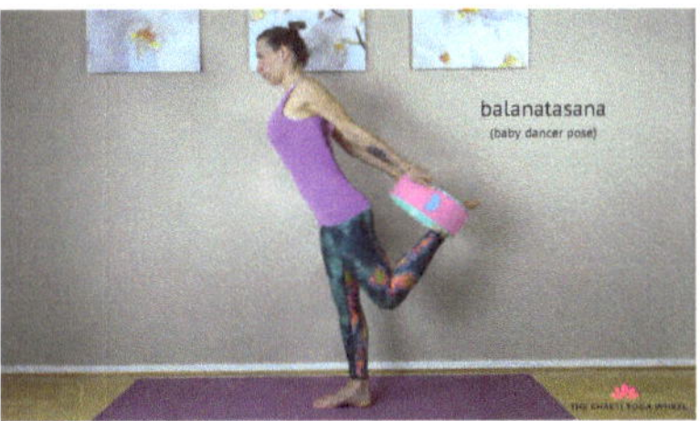

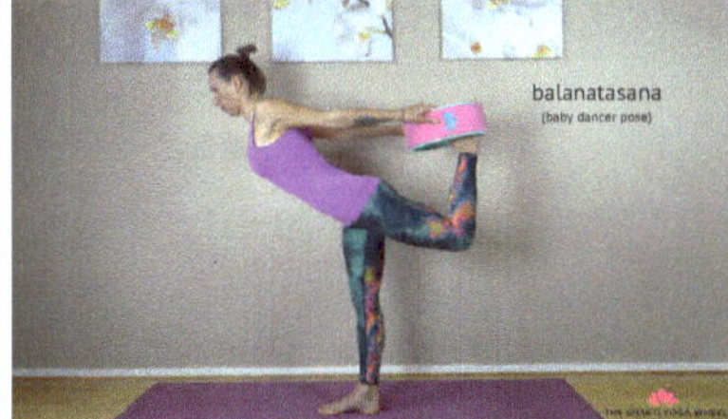

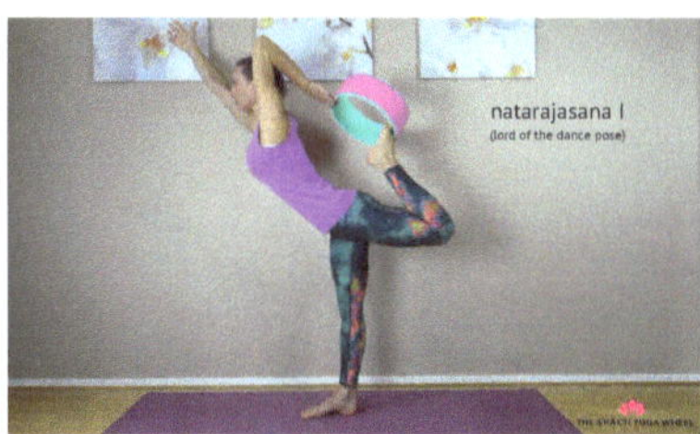

Balanatasana - (baby dancer pose)
Standing firmly on two feet in tadasana, hold the wheel in one hand at the side of your body. Slowly start to bend the same side knee, bringing the heel closer to your seat. Turn your palm so it is facing behind you. Point the foot of the lifted leg and slide it into the wheel. Grab hold of the wheel with the other hand as well. Squeeze the outer edges of the shoulder blades in toward your spine and lift your heart, widening your collarbone. Flex your toes around the wheel and gently kick back with the top of the foot. Keep the knees squeezing in towards each other.

Balanatasana - (baby dancer pose)
If you feel balanced in the previous pose, you could hinge at the hips and send your heart more forward as you kick the foot back and up. Continue to squeeze the knees to midline. Draw energy up from the arch of the standing foot, firm the calf muscle, press the top of the shinbone forward and lift the kneecap.

Natarajasana - (lord of the dance pose)
This pose requires a lot of shoulder mobility as well as balance. If you would like to "flip the grip" begin in tadasana. Hold the wheel in one hand, elbow bent and palm up, as if you were holding a tray. Move your hand slightly behind you. On the same side as you're holding the wheel, bend the knee and point the foot, placing it into the wheel. Draw the head of the armbone further into the shoulder socket and pivot your elbow to the sky. Lift the foot up higher and grab the side of the wheel with your opposite hand as well.

Don't forget the second side!

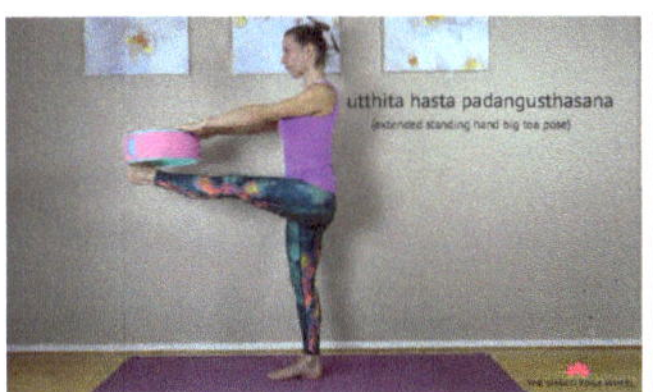

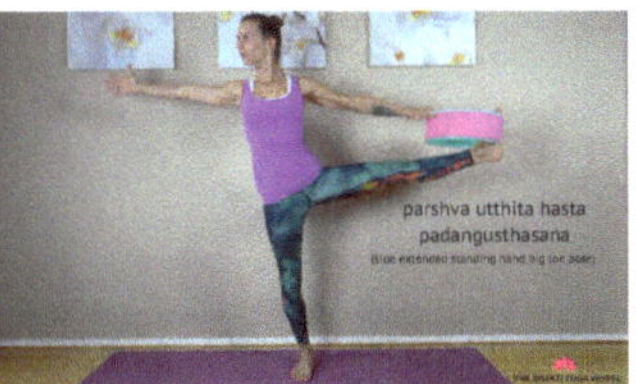

Utthita hasta padangusthasana - (extended standing hand to big toe pose)
From a firm, centered tadasana, hold your wheel in both hands in front of your body. Bend one knee in towards your shin and flex the foot. Press the ball of the foot into the wheel and stand taller, finding length from your hips to your armpits. Hinge forward at the hips and lift your heart. Begin to press the foot forward, extending the lifted leg out in front of you. Keep your standing leg straight and press the top of the thighbone back as you attempt to straighten the lifted the leg.

Parsva utthita hasta padangusthasana - (side extended standing hand to big toe pose)
Press the inner thigh muscles of both legs back and lift your low belly. To extend the lifted leg off to the side, let go of the wheel with your opposite hand and begin to slowly swing the leg to the side. The hand not holding the wheel can come to your hip, or, if balance is steady, that arm can extend out as well.

Don't forget the second side!

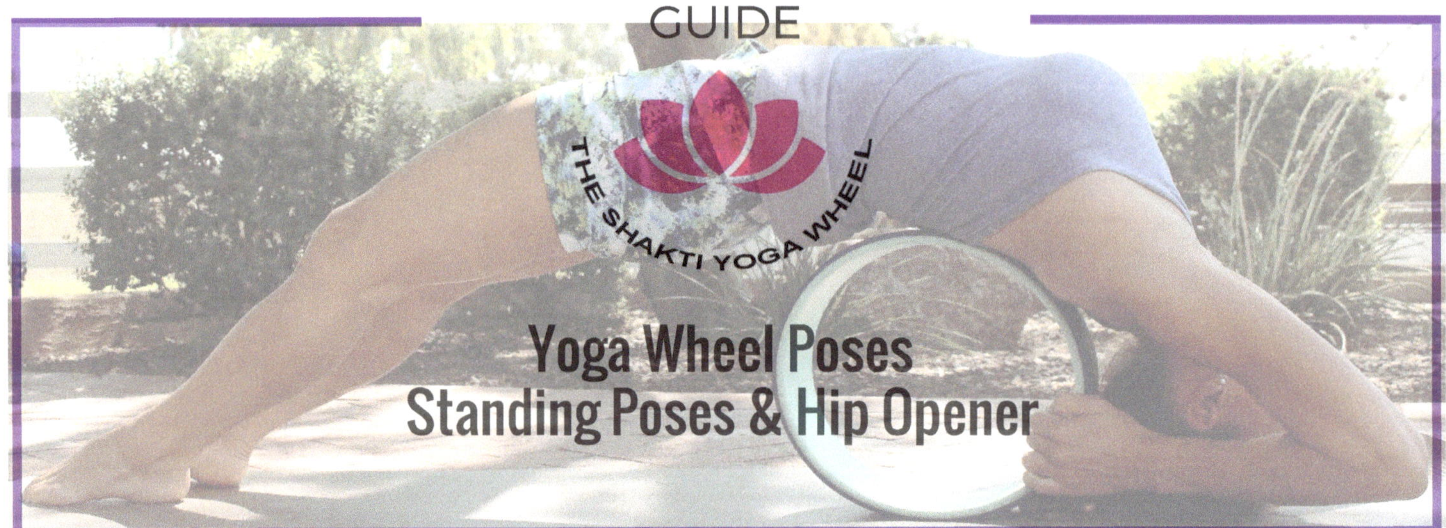

Yoga Wheel Poses
Standing Poses & Hip Opener

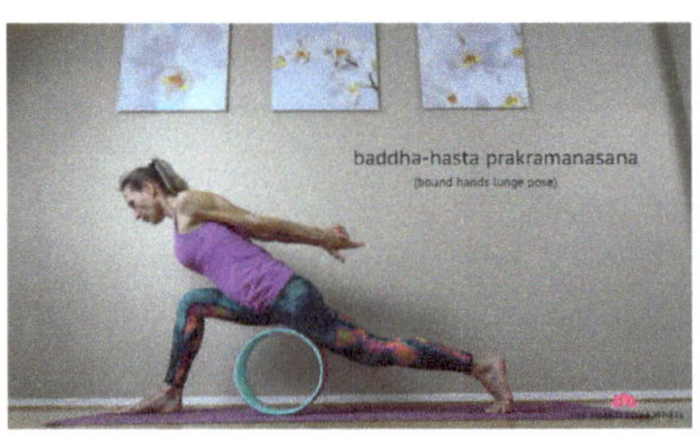

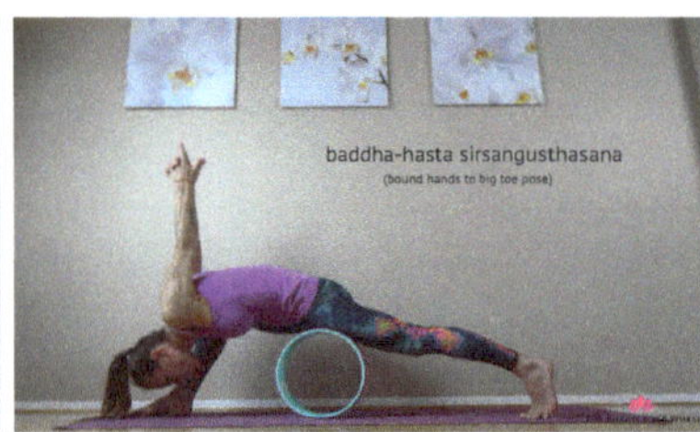

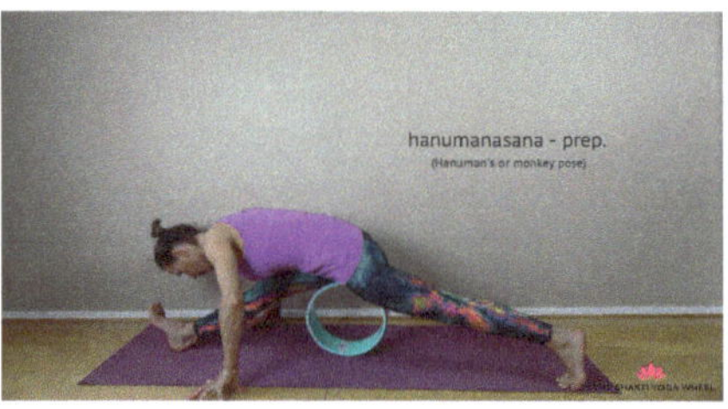

Baddha-hasta prakramansana - (bound lunge pose)
From tadasana, step one leg back into a lunge and place the wheel under the back thighbone. Place the wheel along the thigh wherever it is most comfortable, making sure to keep it above the kneecap. Scissor the hips so that you pull the outer edge of the front hip back and press the outer edge of the back hip forward. Squeeze the feet towards one another and hug the outer hips in. Feeling light on your fingertips, begin to float the arms up and interlace your fingers at your low back. Use the wheel for stability and press the back thighbone into the wheel. Pull your belly up and away from the front thigh. Slightly tuck the chin to the chest, draw the sternum back and roll the heads of the arm bones up and back. Now glide your ears back, lift your heart, and squeeze the outer edges of the shoulder blades together. Visualize the bottom tips of the shoulder blades picking up your heart.

Baddha-hasta sirsangusthasana - (bound hands head to big to toe pose)
Keeping the shoulder blades squeezing toward the spine, begin to bow forward, placing your shoulder on top of your front knee. Drag your front heel back and press the back thighbone into the wheel. Bow deeper, bringing the shoulder now to the inside of the front knee as if you could place your head on the ground near the arch of your front foot.

Hanumanasana prep. - (monkey pose prep.)
Release the hands to the mat. Walk the front foot a few inches forward and begin to straighten the front leg. Roll forward and backward on the wheel, massaging your back thigh muscles as you do so. Keep length in the torso.

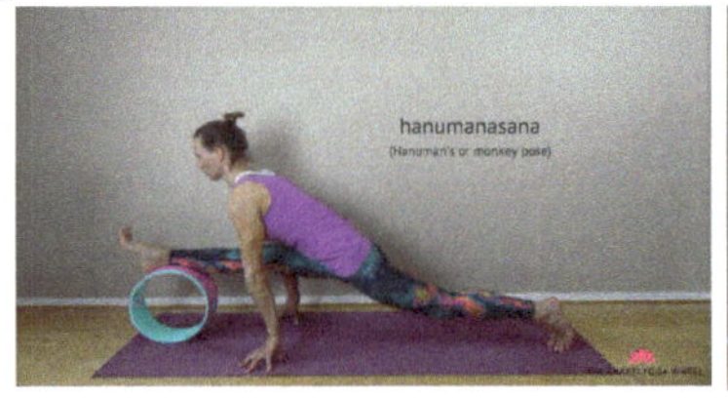

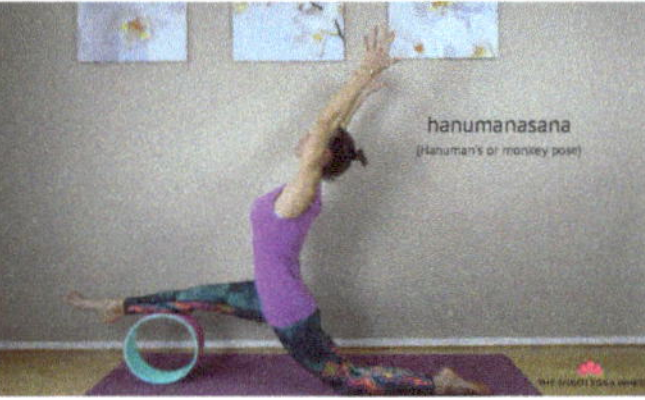

Hanumanasana - (monkey pose)
Drop your back knee and roll the wheel to the front leg to the bottom of the calf muscle. Press your fingertips into the mat. If the ground feels too far away from you, place yoga blocks under your hands to help. Pull the front hip back and press the back hip forward, scissoring the hips to keep them square and level. With the back toes tucked, you may choose to lift the back knee off of the mat, or you can keep the knee planted. Glide the heart more forward as you squeeze the outer edges of the shoulder blades in toward the spine.

Hanumanasana - (monkey pose)
With your back knee on the mat, drag the knee forward as you pull your front outer thigh back and lift the low belly up. With strong, engaged legs, try to float your arms up to the ceiling.

Don't forget the second side!

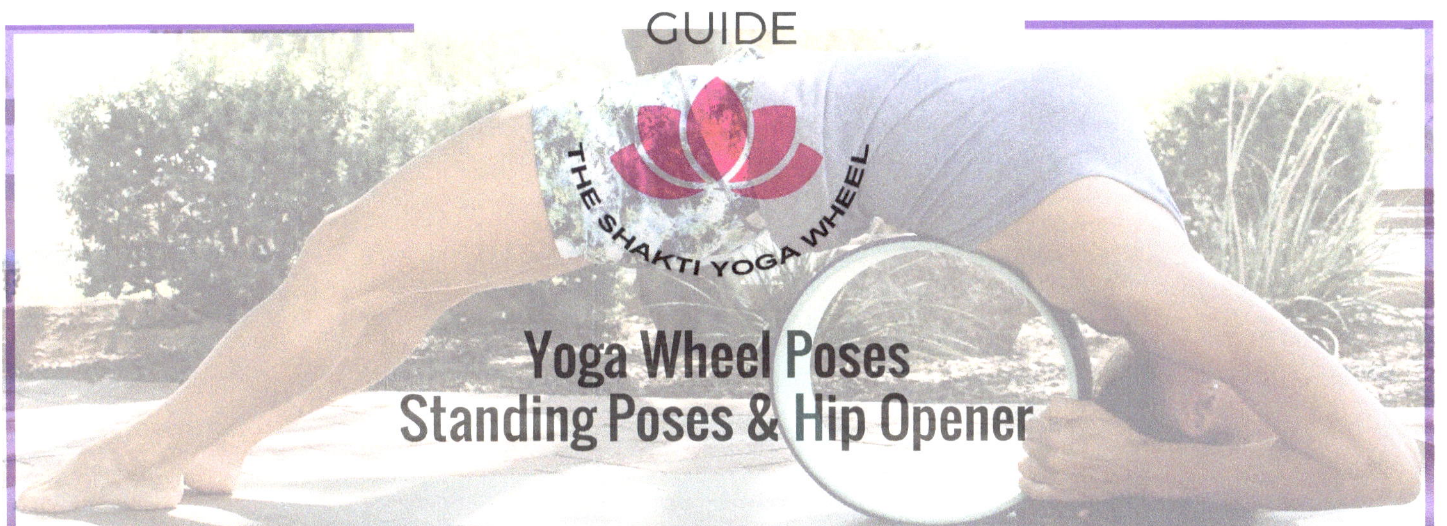

Yoga Wheel Poses
Standing Poses & Hip Opener

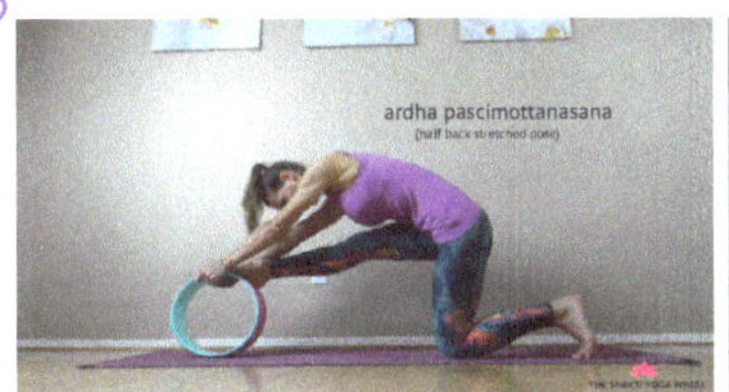

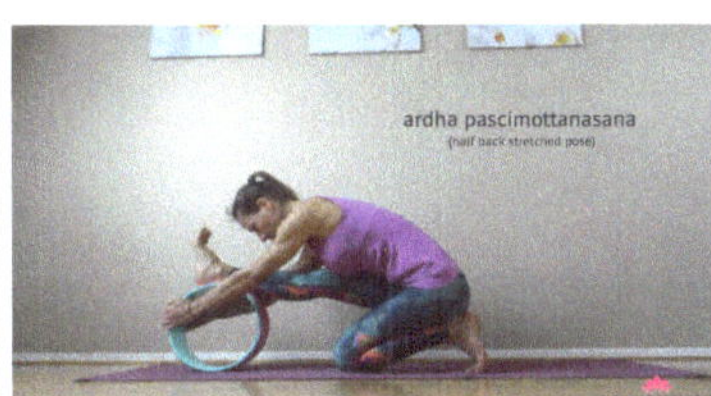

Ardha pascimottanasana - (half back stretched out pose)
Tuck your back toes and bring your hands to the wheel. Shift your hips back so they are directly above the back knee. Place the sole of the front foot on the wheel, point the foot and lengthen your heart forward. Hinge at the top of the thigh and bow over the front leg.

Ardha pascimottanasana - (half back stretched out pose)
To deepen this stretch, roll the wheel an inch or two back and flex the front foot toes back toward the shin, so that the wheel sits just under the Achilles tendon at the bottom of the calf. Walk your hands down the sides of the wheel and bow deeper toward the front shin. Pull the top thigh back and sink the hips down onto the back heel. Bend your elbows to lengthen the spine.

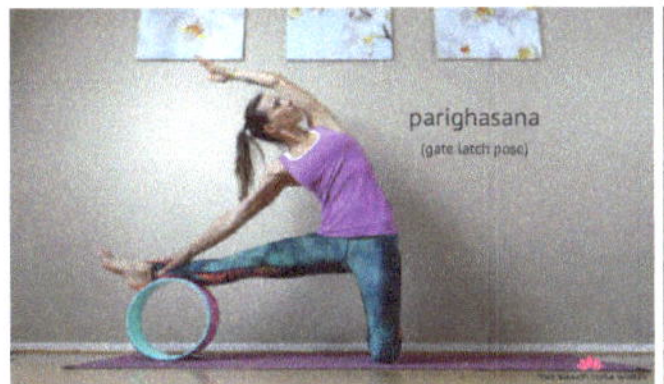

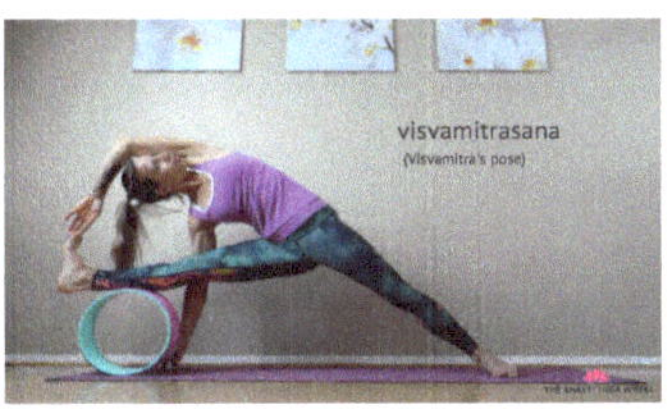

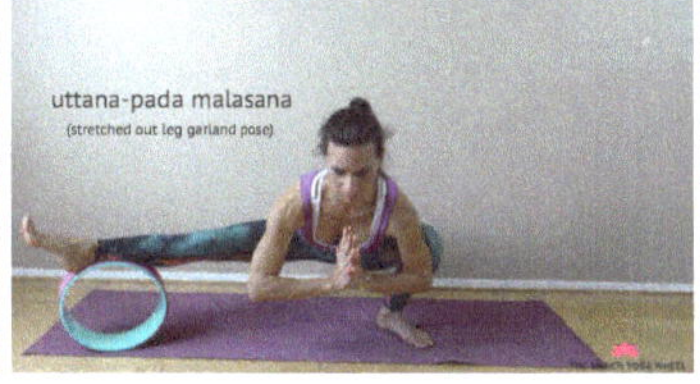

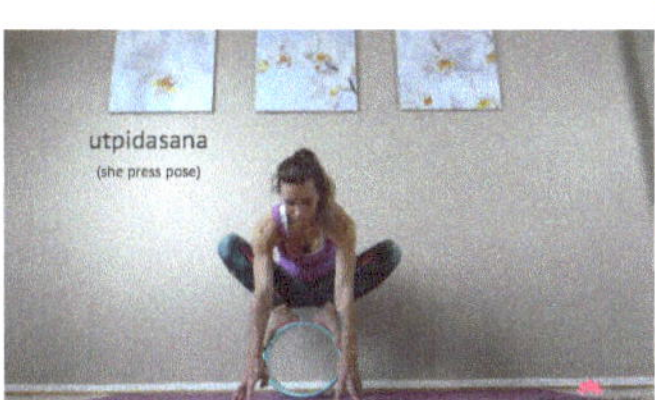

Parighasana - (gate latch pose)
Begin kneeling sideways on your mat, with your hips above the knees and toes tucked if comfortable, for better balance. Extend one leg to the front of your mat and place the wheel under the bottom of the calf as shown. As always, place the wheel where it is most comfortable. Flex, point, or floint the lifted foot to engage the inner thigh muscles. Place one hand on the shin or ankle and side bend toward the wheel. Keep your core engaged as you stretch.

Visvamitrasana - (visvamitra's pose)
From gate pose, bring both hands to the floor on either side of your lifted leg. Tuck the toes of your kneeling leg, and begin to lift your knee off of the mat. Straighten the leg and spin the heel down, bringing the entire sole of the foot to the mat. Bring your top hand to your hip, leaving the bottom hand on the mat outside of the wheel. Press your shinbone into the inside of the upper arm bone to create a strong connection. The final step is to extend the top arm up and over, reaching towards the foot, perhaps grabbing the outer edge of the foot.

Uttana-pada malasana - (stretched out leg garland pose)
Keeping one leg lifted on the wheel, as we did for both gate and visvamitra's pose, we now come into a half squat on the other leg. Bring both hands to the mat in front of you and begin to bend your knee, coming into a squat. Be sure to keep your knee tracking over the middle toe of the planted foot. As you squat, engage your inner thigh muscles and push them back, drawing your inner thighbones deeper into the hip sockets. Continue to flex, point, or floint the lifted foot. You may keep your hand on the mat for help with balance, or bring the hands to prayer in front of your heart space.

Utpidasana - (the press pose)
This is a deep hip opener and is a tricky pose to get in to! You will most likely need to hold on to a chair, a desk or a counter top, or you could stack several large bolsters, one on top of the other for balance. You may even be able to keep your hands on the floor. With your hands on something, you will first step one foot on to the wheel, and then step the other foot up, heels in and the toes pointing out along the sides of the wheel. Both knees are bent deeply. From the inner edges of the feet, pull up to the inner thighs and draw them in, plugging the femur bones deeper into the hip sockets. Although it is a very bent forward posture, press your chest forward and lift up through your heart. For an extra challenge, lift your hands off of the mat/chair/desk/countertop/bolster stack and balance like a circus star!

Don't forget the second side!

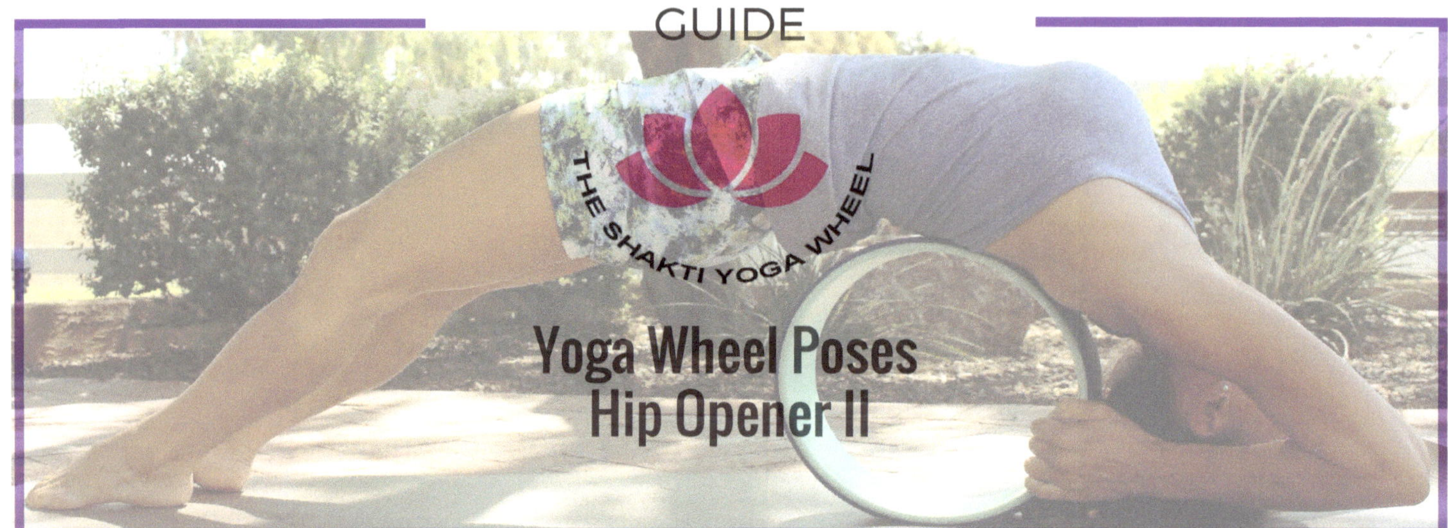

Yoga Wheel Poses
Hip Opener II

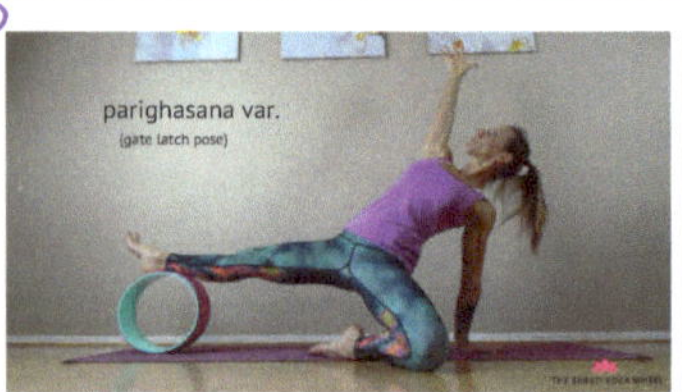
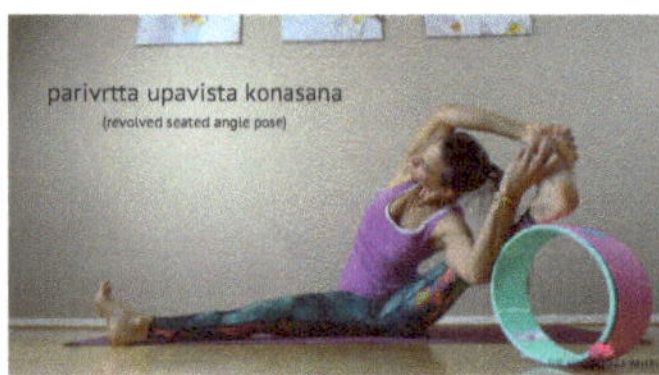
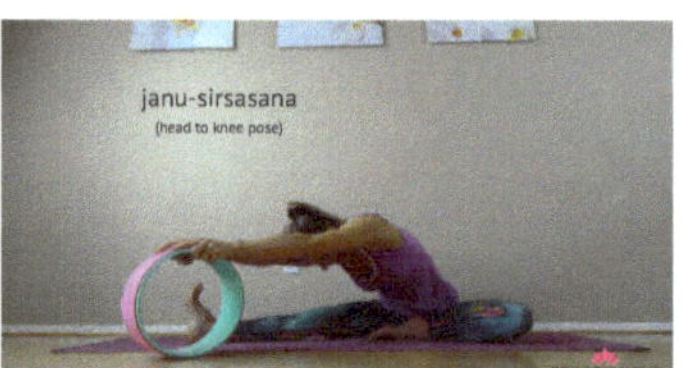
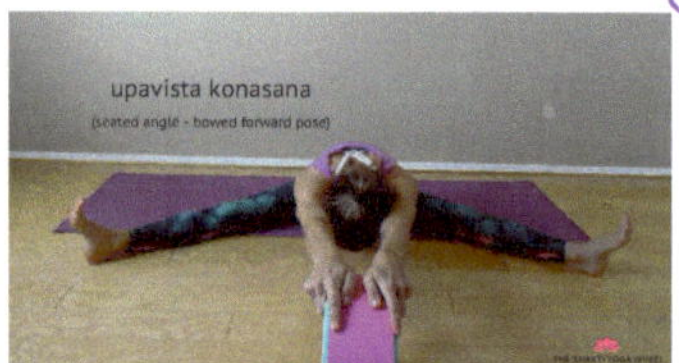

Parighasana variation - (gate latch pose)
Begin is gate pose as you already did. With on leg lifted on the wheel and one leg kneeling on the mat, side bend away from the wheel this time, bringing your fingertips to a block or to the mat beside your bent knee. Draw the ribs down as you lengthen the side of your body.

Parivrtta upavista konasana - (revolved seated angle pose)
From gate pose, come to your seat, keeping the lifted leg where it is on top of the wheel. Straighten the bent leg and open the legs out to a wide angle. Avoid sitting on the low back here. Roll the pelvis more forward so that you can sit on the front of your sit bones. Sitting on a blanket or two will make this easier. Keep your toes and knees pointed to the sky and lift your low belly up. Firm all of the leg muscles to the leg bones and sit taller in your spine. Bring the arm that is closest to the wheel along the inside of the lifted leg, other hand on the hip. Begin to side bend toward the lifted foot, eventually bringing both hands to grab the lifted foot. Look up and under your top armpit, rotating the ribs more to the sky.

Janu-sirsasana - (head to knee pose)
Release the wheel from underneath the leg and bring it in front of you. Bend one knee so that the heel touches the top of the same leg's thighbone. Place both hands on the wheel and roll the wheel along the inside of the straight leg. Draw the ribs down and breath into the back of the lungs. Keep the heart and armpits lifted and you stretch.

Upavista konasana - (seated angle pose bowed forward)
Extend both legs out to a wide angle and sit on the front of the sit bones. Note that most of us will do better sitting on a blanket or two in all seated forward fold postures. Flex the toes back toward the shins, engaging the leg muscles, drawing energy in from the arches of the feet. With the wheel in front of you, between your two legs, place your hands on the wheel and slowly begin to roll the wheel away from you. Breathe into the back of the body while you keep a lift in the heart.

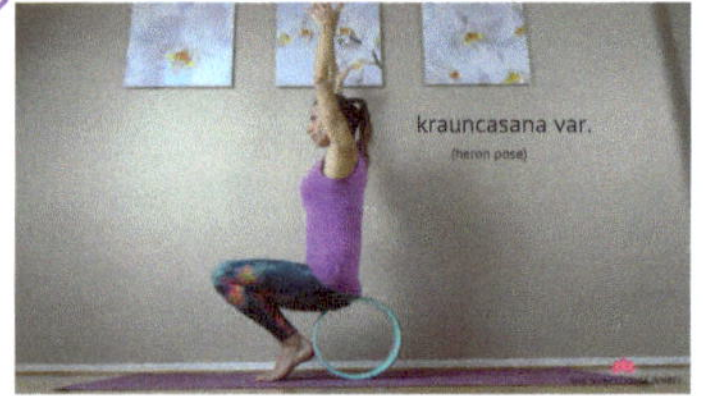
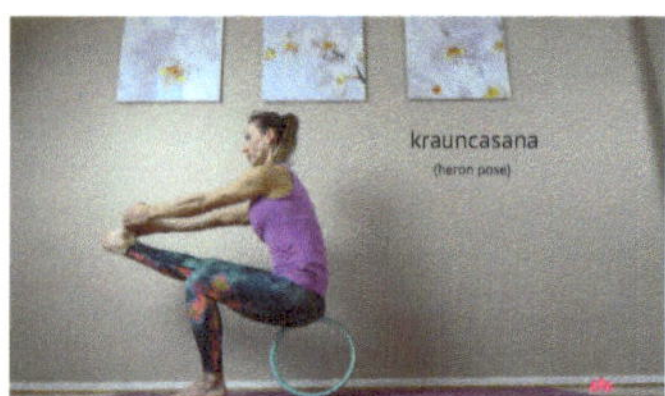
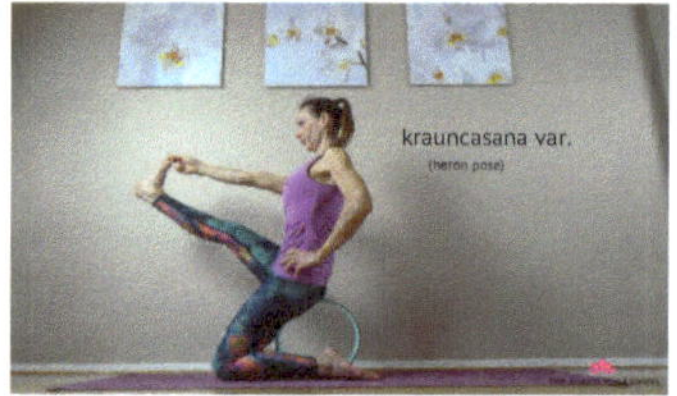
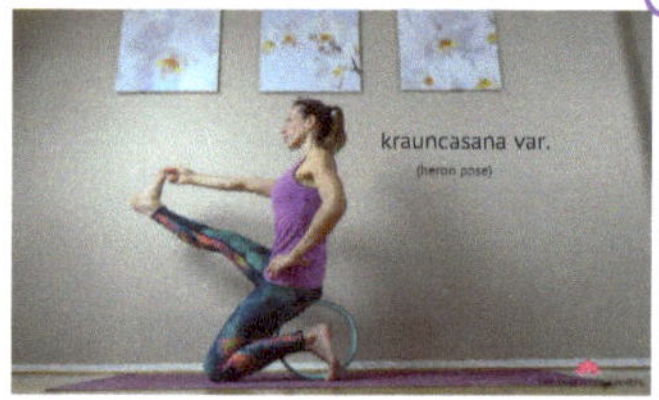

Krauncasana prep. - (heron pose prep)
Sit on the wheel with your inner ankles and inner knees touching. Balance will be harder than you think here. Draw to your midline a lot, by hugging the outer hips in and narrowing the ribs in. Press into the balls of your feet and lift your heels off of the mat. Continue to squeeze the inner ankles together as the heels lift. Draw your ribs down towards your hip points and lift your arms over head.

Krauncasana - (heron pose)
Still sitting on the wheel, lower your arms to your sides and press your heels down. Extend one leg out in front of you and grab hold of the calf, ankle or foot, depending on your hamstring flexibility. Keep length in your spine and avoid rounding the back. Lift the heart as you draw the ribs in and down. Flex the toes of the extended leg back toward the shin and press through the inner heel and big toe mound.

Krauncasana variation - (heron pose variation)
From the previous pose, release your lifted leg back to the floor. Still sitting on the wheel, set up as shown, with one shin on the mat to the outside of the wheel, where the top of the foot is on the mat and the toes are pointing toward the back of the mat. Place one hand on your hip. Extend the other leg out in front of you and grab hold of the big toe with the peace fingers of the same side hand. Lift your low belly and lengthen your spine.

Krauncasana variation - (heron pose variation)
Set up the same way as in the previous photo, only this time, the bottom leg toes will be tucked, rather than the top of the foot flat to the mat.

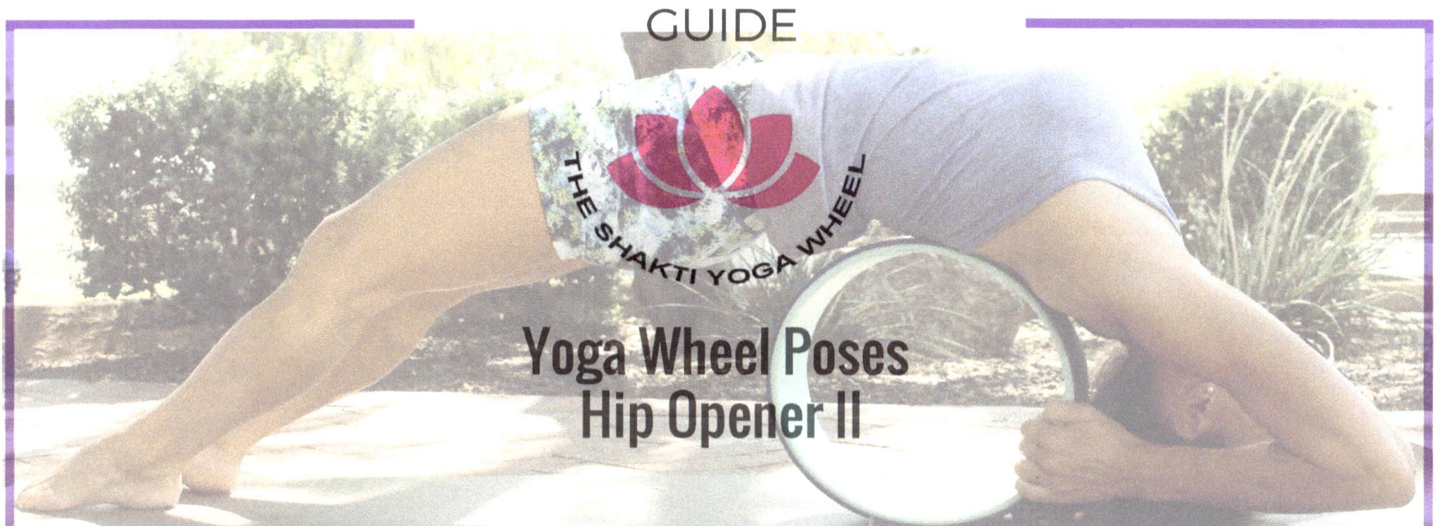

Yoga Wheel Poses
Hip Opener II

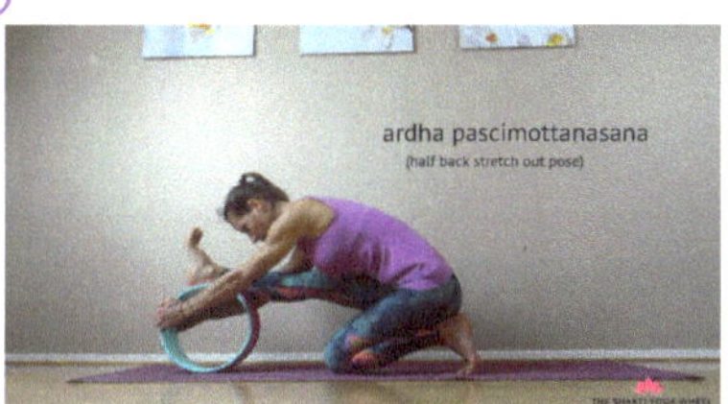

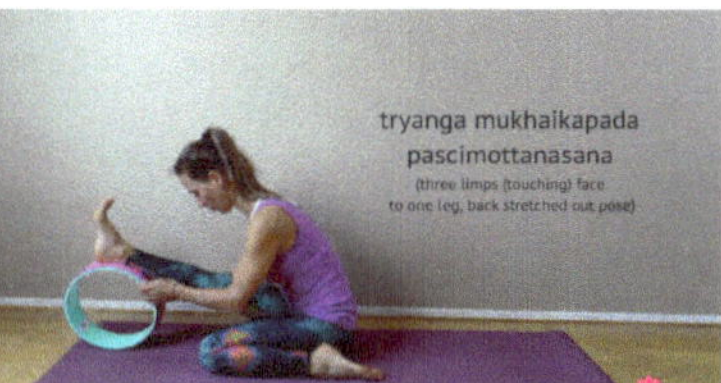

Ardha pascimottanasana - (half back stretched out pose)
Release the lifted leg back to the mat and press into your feet to lift your seat off of the wheel. Roll the wheel forward and place it under the Achilles tendon/bottom of the calf your forward leg. Walk your hands down the sides of the wheel and bow deeper toward the front shin. Flex the toes in toward the shin. Pull the top thigh back and sink the hips down onto the back heel. Bend your elbows to lengthen the spine.

Tryanga mukhaikapada pascimottanasan - (three limbs face to one leg back stretched out pose)
From the previous pose, un-tuck your toes and come to the top of the foot for ardha virasana (half hero pose). Bring your seat to the mat. If it is not possible to sit all the way down without knee pain, sit on a blanket or a block. Keep the foot and ankle active by flicking all five toes into the mat. Your forward leg will be lifted on the wheel. Engage all the muscles of the leg to the leg bones and fold over the extended leg.

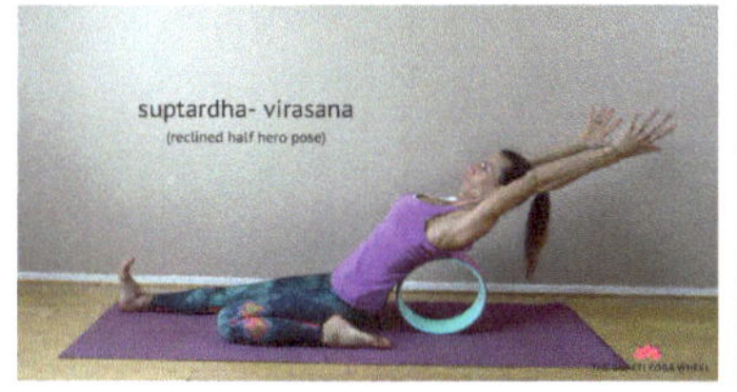

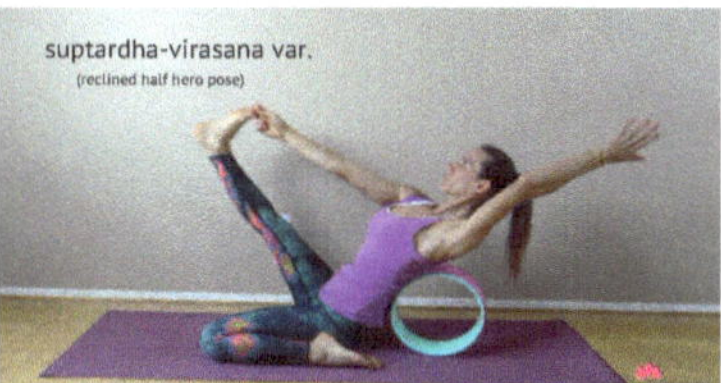

Suptardha-virasana - (reclined half hero pose)
Keep the position of the legs but move the wheel out from under your front leg behind you to your spine. Reach your arms up overhead and gently backbend over the wheel. As the arms lift up, the ribs will widen and stick out. Continue to narrow the ribs even as you lift your arms up and draw the ribs down as you curl into the backbend.

Suptardha-virasana variation - (reclined half hero pose variation)
From the previous pose, if you'd like to add a hamstring stretch to it, simply lift the straight leg up and grab hold of the big toe with your peace fingers. From the inner edge of the foot, draw energy up to the inner thigh and lift the low belly.

Don't forget the second side!

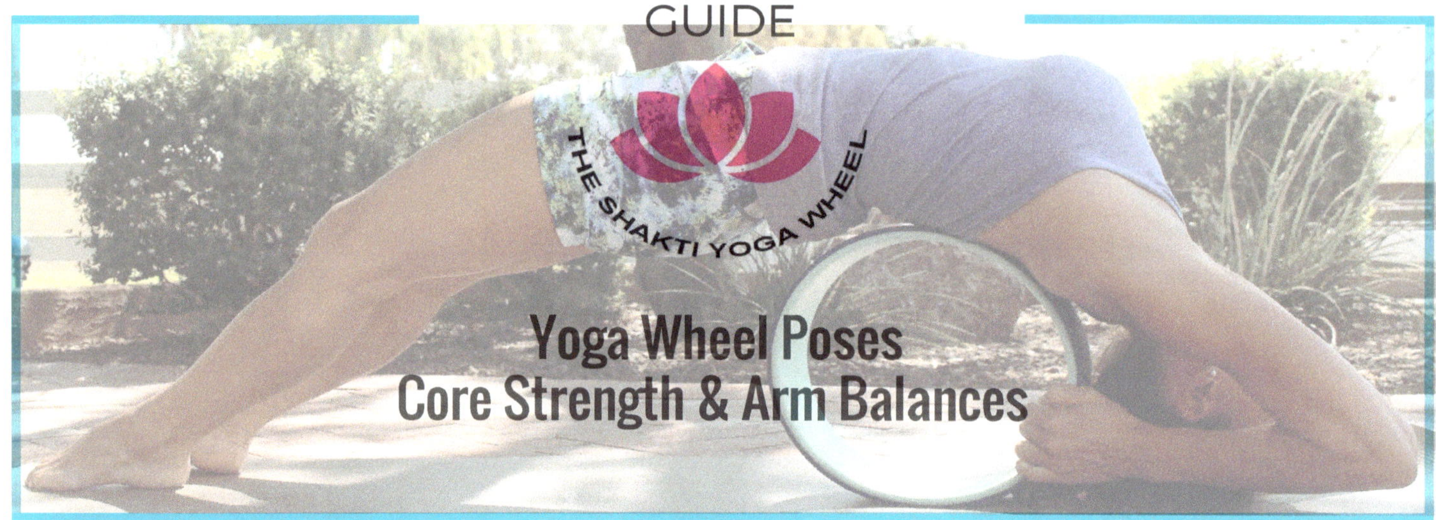

Yoga Wheel Poses
Core Strength & Arm Balances

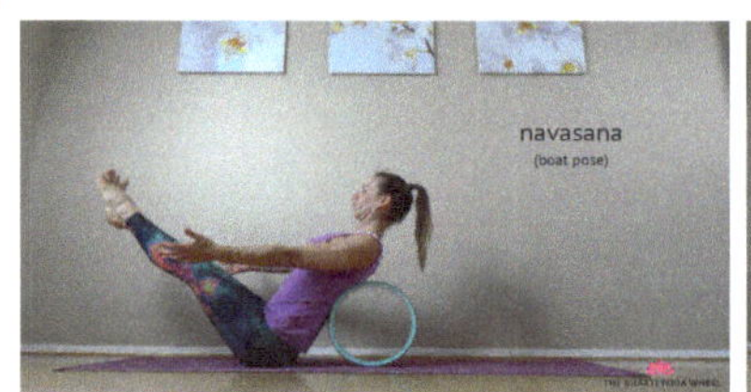

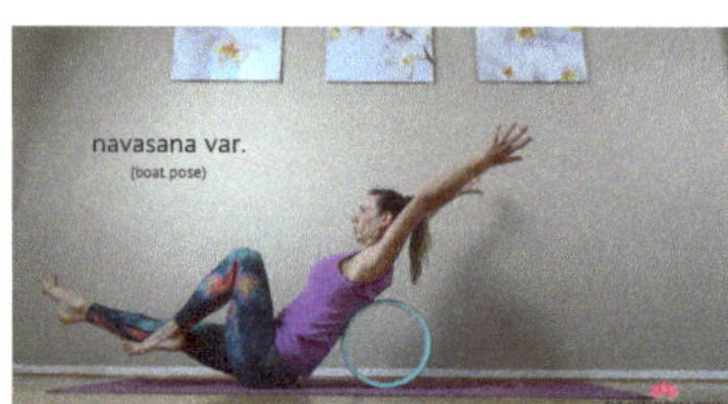

Navasana - (boat pose)

Come to a seat and place the wheel behind you, in line with your spine. Bend your knees in front of you, feet flat on the mat, and squeeze your inner knees together. Grab the backs of your thighs and start to lean back, lifting your heels off of the mat and extending your heart up. The wheel will be most helpful along the upper back, at the base of your shoulder blades, however, experiment with the placement of the wheel and see what feels best for you. Engage your core and lift your toes off of the mat. From here you can lift your shins so they are parallel with the floor. Then you could let go of the backs of your thighs and reach your arms out in front of you. Finally you will extend the legs straight. Hold for five full breaths.

Navasana variation - (boat pose variation)

Draw your ribs in towards each other and down towards the hip points as you reach your arms over head. Bend one knee and hold the pose for five full breaths. Switch legs..

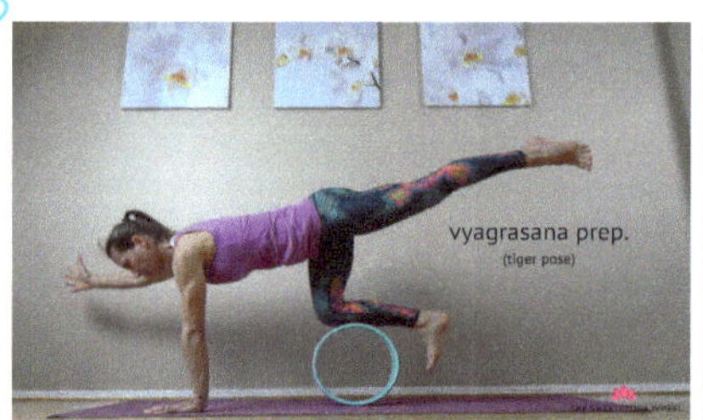

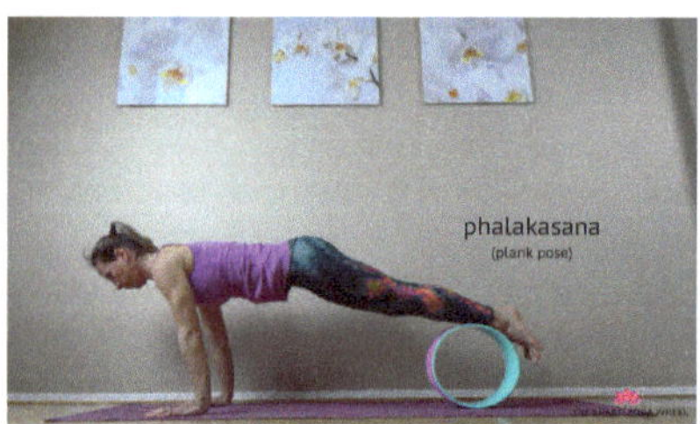

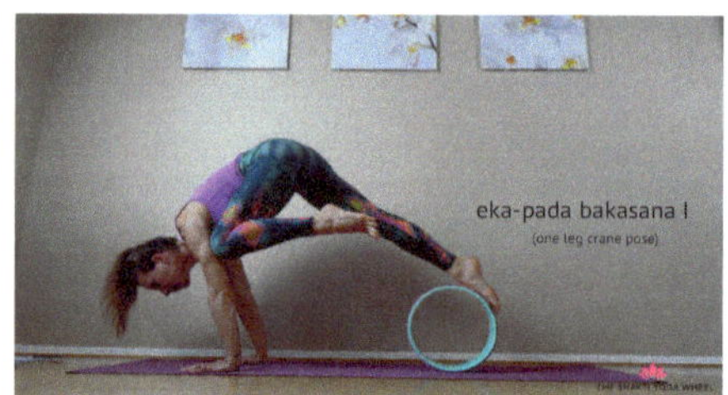

Vyaghrasana preparation - (tiger pose prep.)
From hands and knees, tuck the toes and press up into downward facing dog. Roll the wheel towards your feet, lift one leg, and place that shin on top of the wheel just below the knee, at the top of the shinbone. Flex the foot of that leg strongly. Hug to the midline by firming the forearms in towards each other and engaging the inner thigh muscles. Press into your palms, draw both sides of the waistline back and see if you can lift your planted downward dog foot off of the mat. Reach the arm that is the same side as where you have the wheel out in front of you, bicep in line with the ear.

Phalakasana - (plank pose)
Begin on hands and knees. Lift one foot towards your seat as if you would kick yourself in the butt. Place the wheel along the bottom of the shinbone. Do the same with the other leg. Your feet will be side by side on the wheel. Press into your palms and draw the front ribs in toward each other and back toward the spine. Lift your knees off of the mat and roll the wheel away from you, extending the legs straight. At the top of a push-up, with your shoulders directly over the wrists, hug your forearms in towards each other. Lengthen out through the top of your head.

Eka-pada bakasana - (one leg crane pose)
Draw the navel to the spine and press the inner thighs up, piking the hips up to the sky. Roll slightly forward so your shoulders are just past your wrists. Lift one leg off of the wheel and hug the knee into the back of the triceps. Press the knee and upper arm bone into one another for strength. Press into your palms and draw the waistline back.

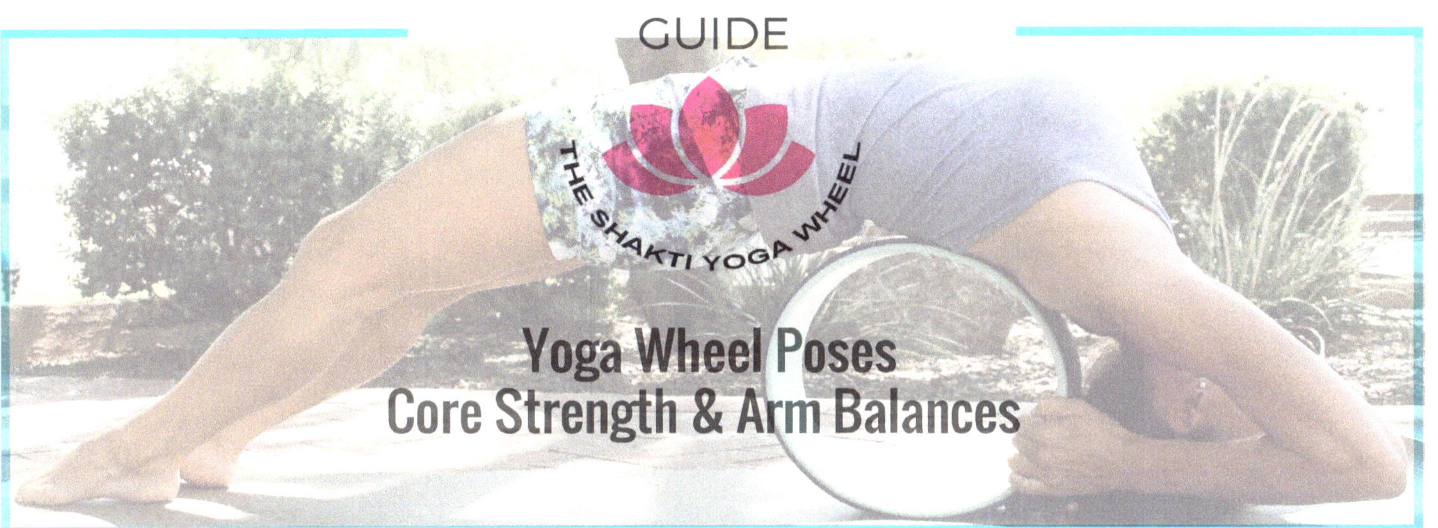

Yoga Wheel Poses
Core Strength & Arm Balances

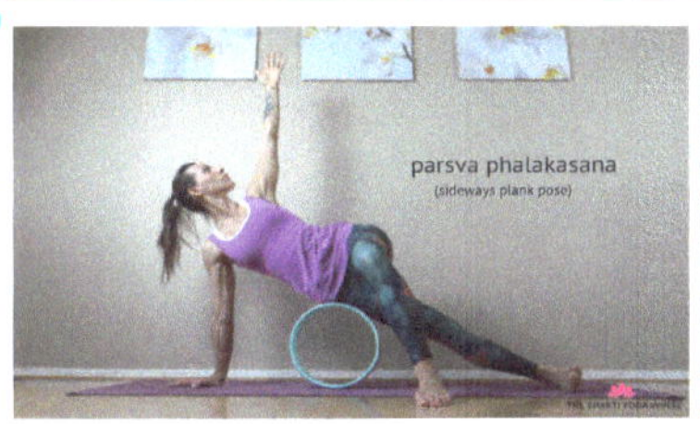

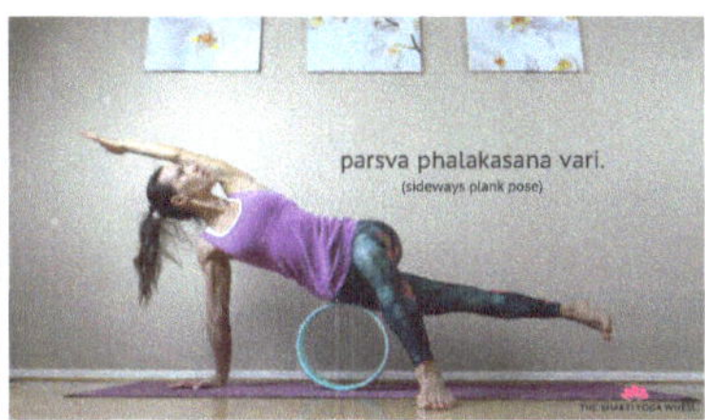

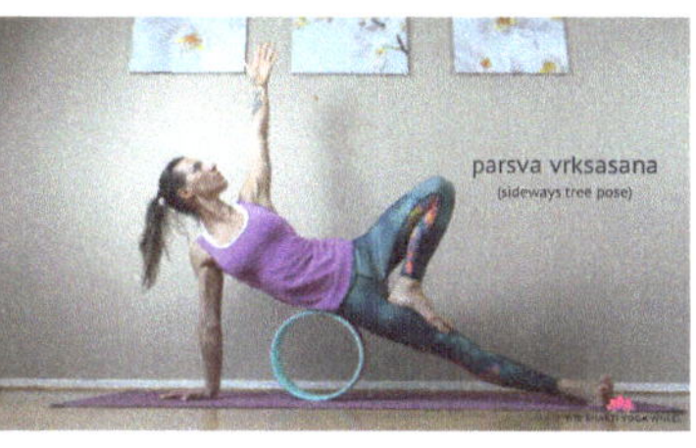

Parsva phalankasana - (sideways plank pose)
Come into a side plank. Bend the top leg and step the sole of the foot in front of the straight bottom leg. Flex the toes of the bottom foot back toward the shin to maintain a strong and square ankle. Slide the wheel underneath the outer thigh of the straight bottom leg. Experiment with the placement of the wheel, as there may be some sensitive spots on the outer thigh along the IT band where you may or may not want the wheel pressing into. Press into your foundation, engage the inner thigh muscles and draw the ribs in. Root into your planted palm and draw the shoulder blades down the back. Extend out in all directions.

Parsva phalankasana variation- (sideways plank pose)
If you feel stable in the previous pose, extend the top arm overhead, bicep in line with your ear. Lengthen through that top arm so much that he bottom foot lifts off of the mat.

Parsva vksasana - (sideways plank pose)
To practice with a tree pose variation in side plank, press the pinky toe side of the bottom foot into the mat. Keep that ankle strong and square and lift top leg up, pressing the sole of the foot into the inner thigh of the straight bottom leg. Extend your top arm toward the sky.

Don't forget the second side!

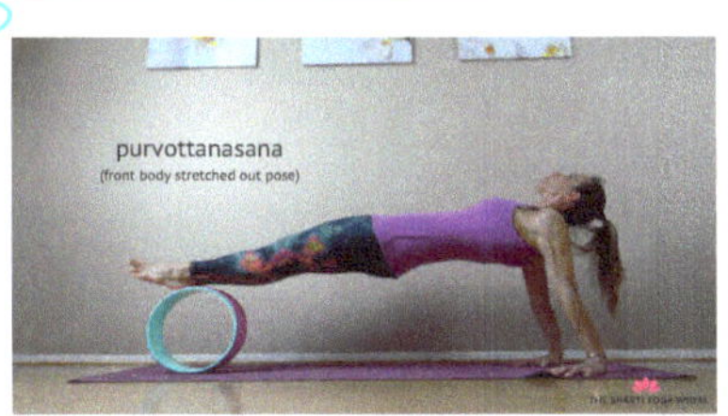

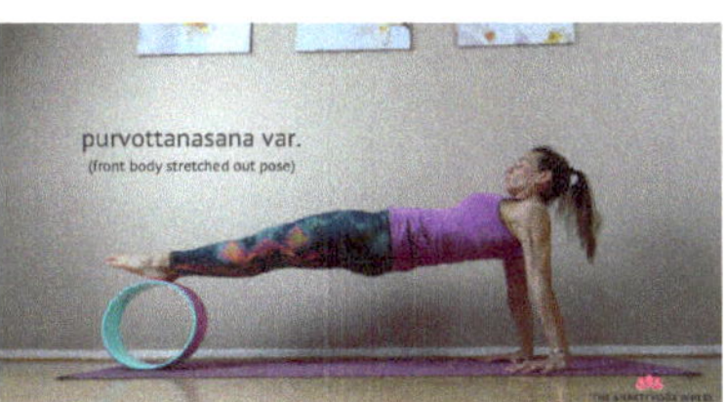

Purvottanasana - (front body stretched out pose)
Begin seated with your legs bent in front of you. Lift up one foot at a time and place the wheel under the soles of your feet. Place your hands on your mat behind you, fingertips pointing in towards your seat. Press the inner edges of your hands down and lift your heart up. Narrow your ribs and squeeze the inner thighs together. Lift your belly up and lift your seat off of the mat. Roll the wheel away from you to straighten your legs. Gaze upward or back if your neck feels okay this way. Reach out through the balls of your feet.

Purvottanasana variation - (front body stretched out pose)
Keep the same shape of the previous pose, but for this variation, you will tuck your chin and look towards your belly button. Draw the ribs in and down.

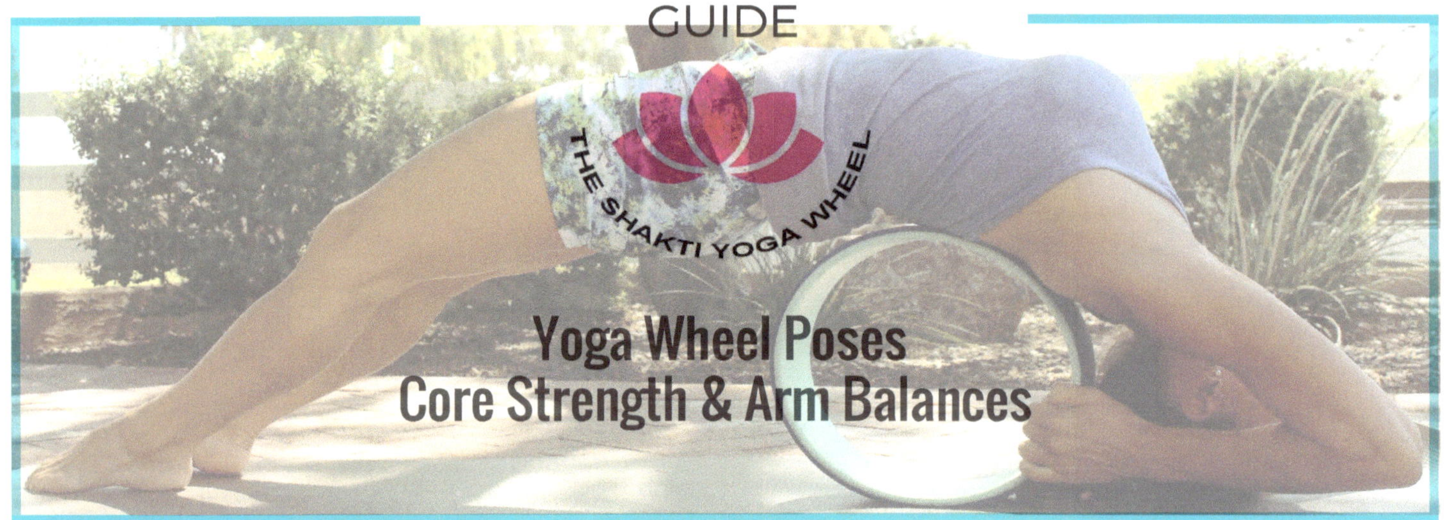

Yoga Wheel Poses
Core Strength & Arm Balances

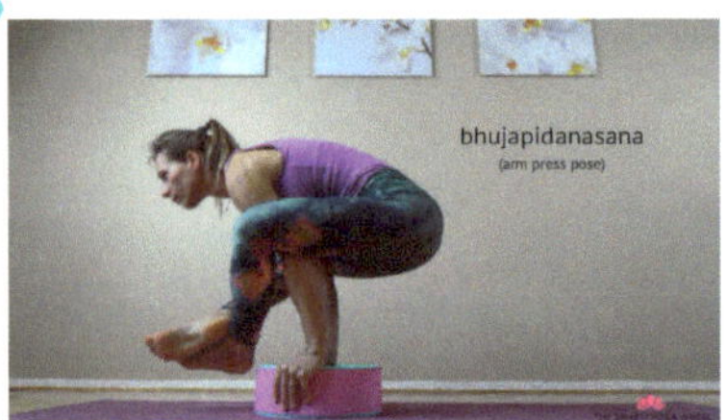

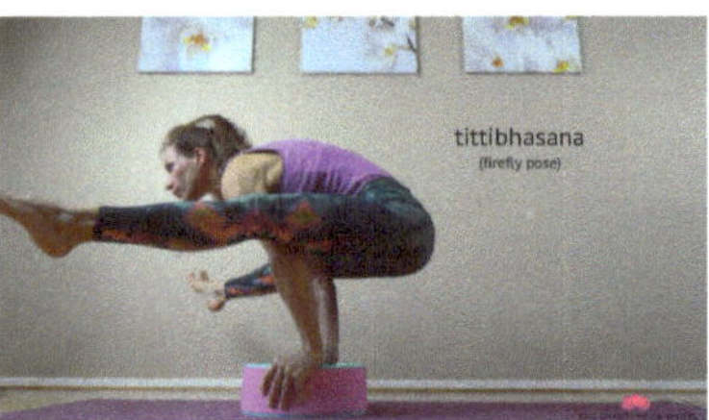

Bhujapidasana - (arm pressure pose)
For this pose, turn the wheel onto its side. Come to standing in front of the wheel with your feet as wide as your mat. Lift and spread your toes, drawing energy up from the arches of your feet to your low belly. Bend your knees and squat, reaching your hands down between your legs. Press your inner thighs back. Grab your right calf muscle with your hand and press the calf forward, working your shoulder under the back of the thigh as much as possible. Do the same on the left. Continue to wiggle your arms under your thighs and grab onto the sides of yoga wheel. Squeeze your inner thighs into your upper arm bones and pull the navel back to the spine. Wiggle your toes slightly forward and then cross one ankle in front of the other. Flex your feet and pull the feet against one another. On an inhale, lift your feet off the mat.

Tittibhasana - (firefly pose)
Continue to squeeze the inner thighs into the upper arm bones. Now begin to extend your legs straight. Reach out through active toes and lift your heart. Keep the inner edge of your hands rooted.

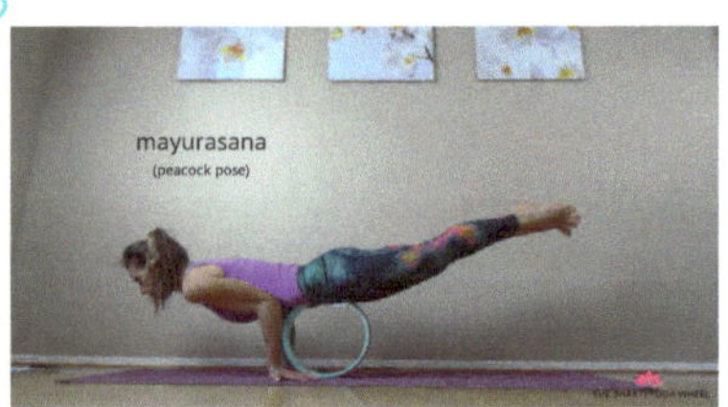

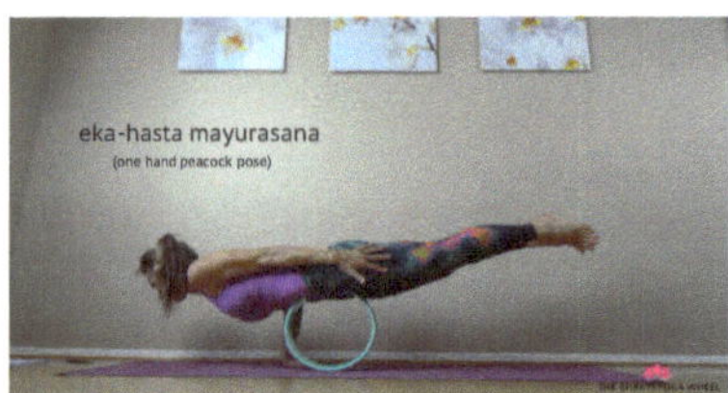

Mayurasana - (peacock pose)
Kneel down and place the wheel in front of you, between your thighs. Lean over the wheel so that your low belly rests atop the wheel. Lengthen your spine. Turn your fingertips to point to the back of the mat, and press the entire palm to the mat, so your forearms are forward. Squeeze your elbows into your sides. Play with extending the heart forward so much that the legs behind you can extend and lift up off of the mat.

Eka-hasta mayurasana - (one hand peacock pose)
If you feel okay in the previous pose, reach one hand back and press your arm along the outer thigh.

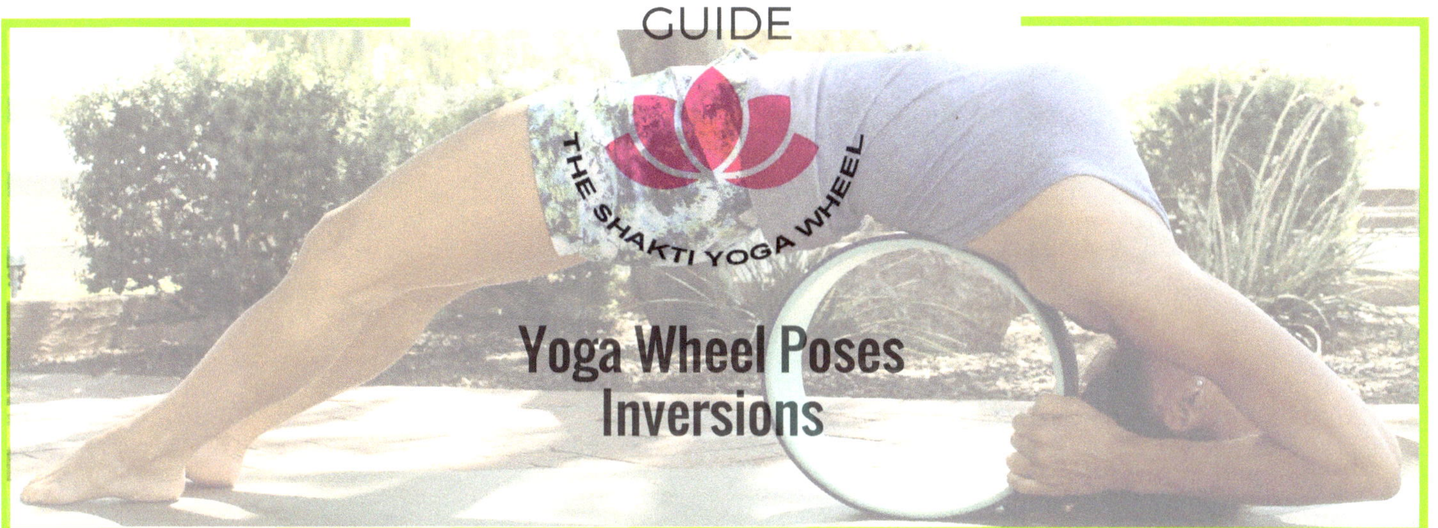

Yoga Wheel Poses
Inversions

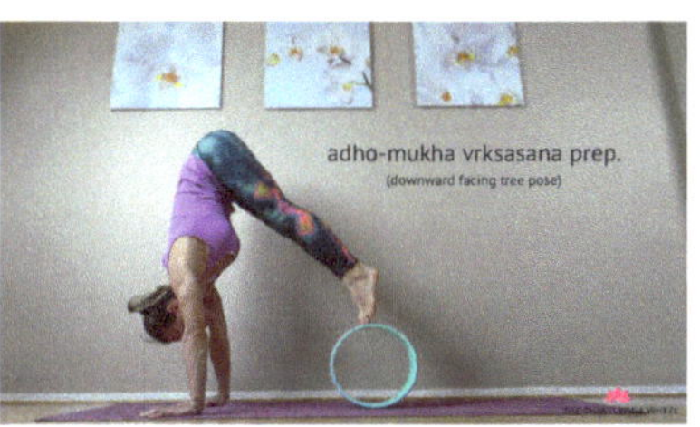
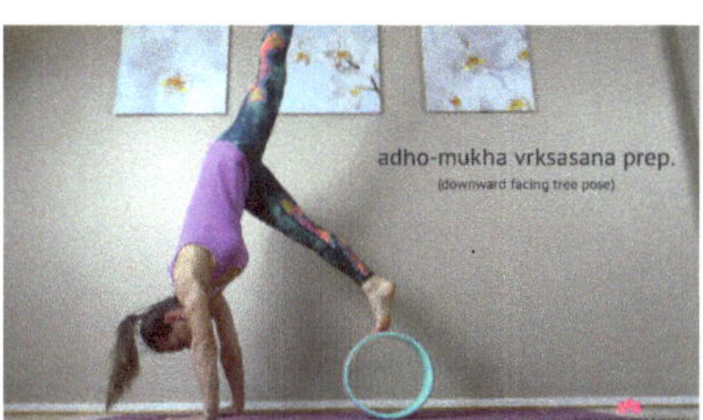

Ado-mukha vrksasana preperation - (downward facing tree pose prep.)
Begin in plank pose, with your shoulders directly over your wrists and the tops of your feet on the wheel, (see "phlankasana" page 4). Push firmly into your hands and draw the navel to the spine. Squeeze your hands and your feet toward each other and lift your hips to the sky. Press into the tops of the feet as you roll the wheel toward the front of the mat, stacking hips over shoulders over wrists.

You can stay on the tops of your feet, lifting the hips high, or you can curl the toes under and press into the balls of your feet. Continue to draw the navel to the spine. Firm the lowest part of the belly in and up. Roll between plank pose and this handstand preparation several times to gain strength and stability. Make sure the inner edges of your hands stay connected to the mat.

Ado-mukha vrksasana preparation - (downward facing tree pose prep.)
Once you feel strong in the previous pose, you are ready to play with lifting one leg. Claw the fingertips into the mat and pull energy from the palms up the arms to the heart center. Draw the ribs down toward the hip creases and lift the hip creases toward the ribs. Firm the muscles of the legs and begin to lift one foot off of the wheel. Reach up through the ball of the lifted foot.

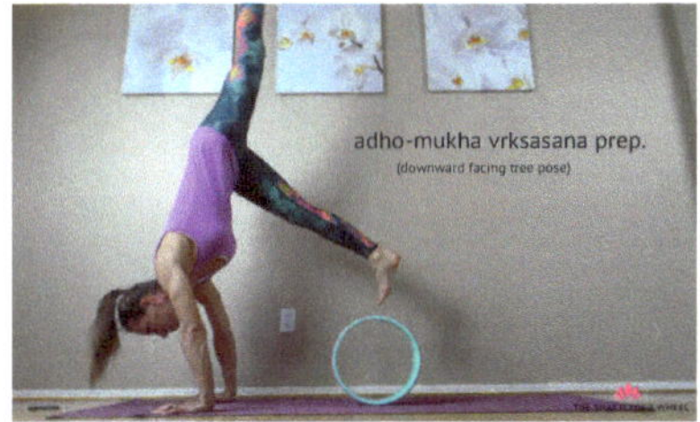
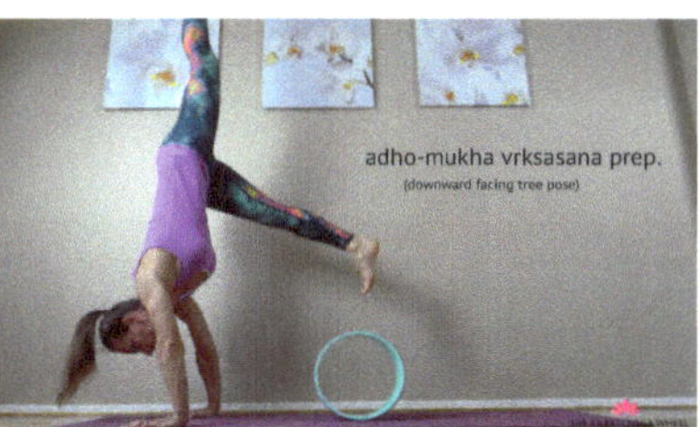

Ado-mukha vrksasana preperation - (downward facing tree pose prep.)
With one leg extended into your handstand, it is time to work on lifting the second leg. Pull the wheel towards the hands and shift the hips back over the shoulders. Hug the ribs in. Firm the entire belly to the spine and then lift the belly up. Squeeze the outer hips in and try to lift the second foot off of the wheel.

Ado-mukha vrksasana preparation - (downward facing tree pose prep.)
Keep your arms firm. It is paramount that as you transition weight onto your hands, you lift up through the inner left thigh (as opposed to reaching the left leg behind you). Draw the low belly in to support the pelvis. Do not aim to get your legs overhead; instead, aim to place your pelvis over your chest and shoulders. When you lead with your legs and not your pelvis, you will often backbend and find balance elusive. Eventually, you will be able to bring the right leg parallel to the floor into an inverted Utthita Hasta Padangusthasana. At this stage, don't lift the right leg higher—it will serve as an anchor and keep you from flipping over. Once you have the right leg parallel to the floor, internally rotate the thighs, drawing them energetically into the midline. Your legs should feel like scissor blades: bolted firmly into their common point (the pelvis) and moving along, but not away from, the midline.

Once you have found balance, draw your legs together. Push down into the hands and actively reach up through the feet and legs. As you hug your legs into the midline, move the tailbone and the tops of the buttocks toward your heels. This will introduce length to the lumbar spine. Draw your low ribs toward the frontal hipbones to prevent any backbending. Make your body feel like an inverted Urdhva Hastasana. Grow even taller by reaching your legs strongly up and away from your rooted and stable palms.

Try to gently land back on your yoga wheel. Practice the transitions. Do both legs!

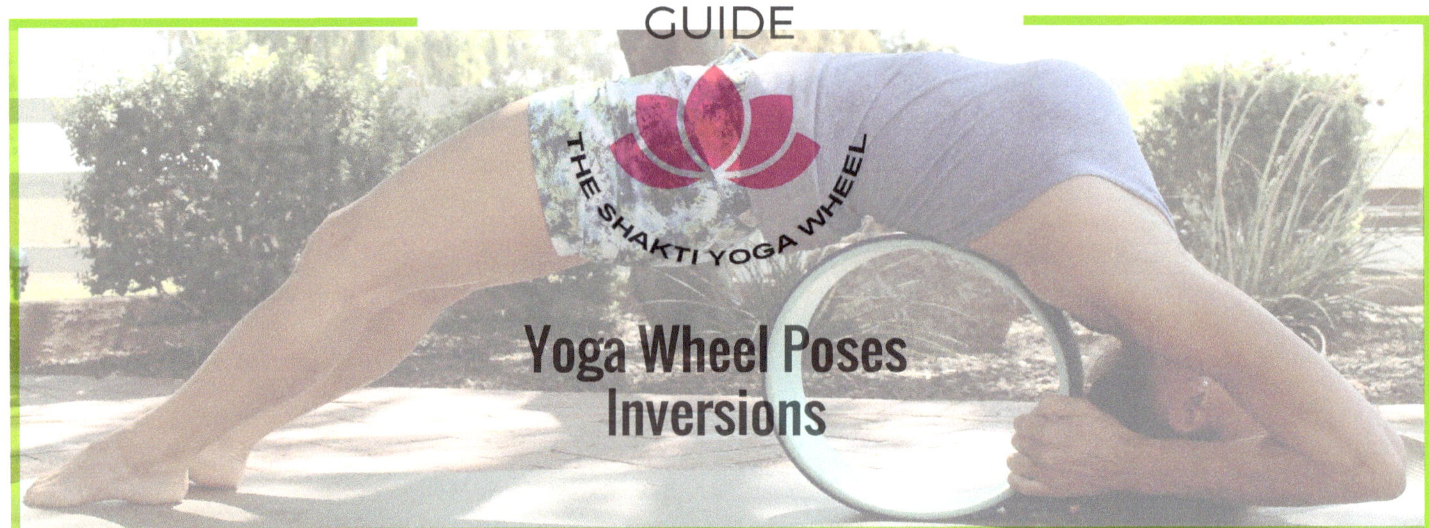

Yoga Wheel Poses
Inversions

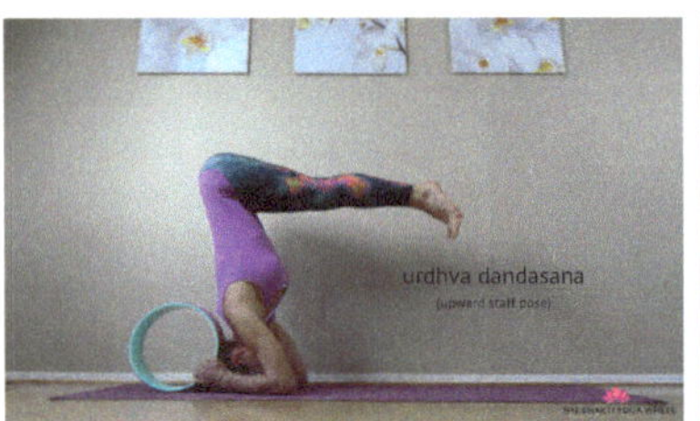

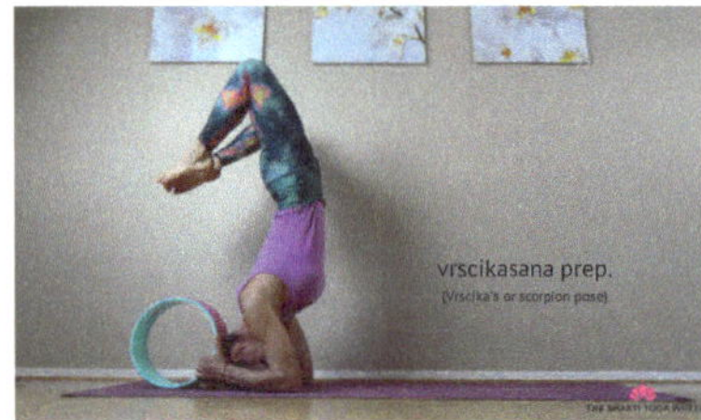

Urdhva dandasana to sirsasana I (upward staff pose to supported headstand I)
Begin on hands and knees. Lengthen your side body and then come down to your forearms, holding the wheel between your palms, thumbs pointing up. Melt the heart toward the mat and invite the arm bones to sink deeper into the shoulder the sockets. Firm the belly to the spine. Release the top of the head to the mat, and press the back of the skull into the wheel. Slide your shoulder blades towards the waistline. Tuck your toes and lift your knees off of the mat, hips high like downward facing dog. Walk your feet in closer to your elbows.

Press into your toes, shift your hips over the shoulders and lift one foot at a time, (or both at the same time), to hip height. Strongly root the forearms into the mat. From here, you could lift the toes to the sky and come into sirsasana I, supported headstand. When you do this, lengthen out through the balls of the feet.

Vrscikasana I - (scorpion pose)
From the previous pose, bend your knees and point your feet toward your head. Continue to use the wheel for support by pressing your head into the wheel and the wheel into your head. Draw the bottom edges of the shoulder blades together and then down the back towards your waistline. Squeeze the inner knees in.

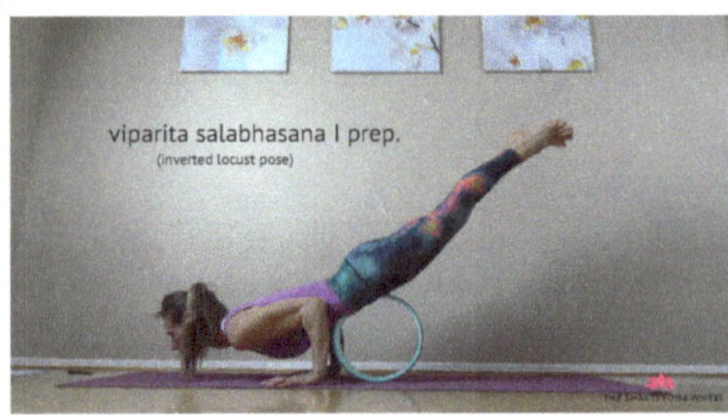

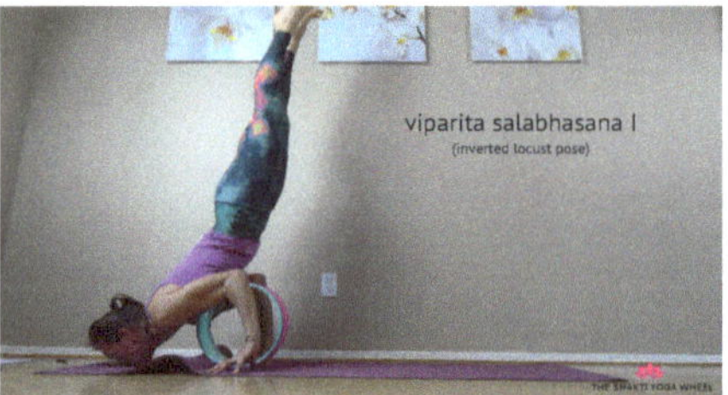

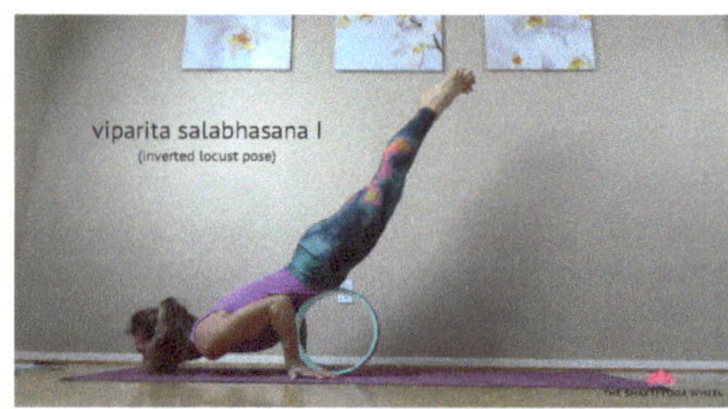

Viparita salabhasana I preparation - (locust pose prep.)
Kneel on the mat with the wheel placed between the thighs. Tuck your toes and lean your torso forward into the wheel. (See "back and abdominal strength" on page 1). Place your palms on the mat. Bend the elbows and squeeze them into the sides of the body. Broaden the collarbone by taking the head of the arm bones back. Bring the chin closer to the mat, lift the knees up and walk the legs back until they are straight. Squeeze the shoulder blades together and press the heart forward. Lengthen through the heart so much that your feet lift off of the mat.

Viparita salabhasana I preparation - (locust pose prep.)
From the previous pose, walk the hands back a few inches and bring your chin all the way to the mat. Squeeze the legs toward each other and lift them higher to the sky.

Viparita salabhasana I preparation - (locust pose prep.)
For this variation, you will turn your hands around, pointing the fingertips toward the back of the mat. Continue to hug to your midline.

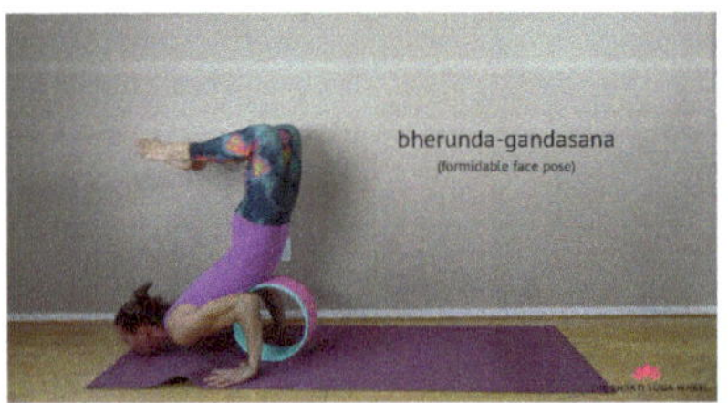

Bherunda-gandasana - (formidable face pose)
Place your palms as they were for the first variation of locust, just as they would be for plank pose or for a push up. Press the palms into the mat and firm the shoulders away from the ears. With your legs extended to the sky, bend your knees, pointing your toes toward your head..

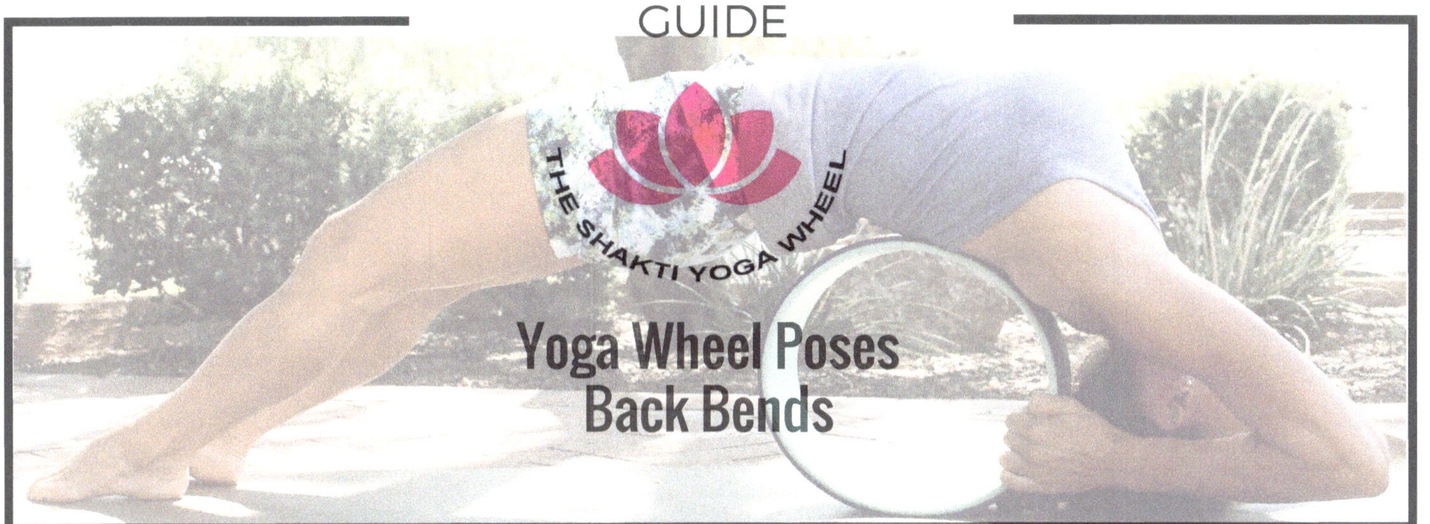

Yoga Wheel Poses
Back Bends

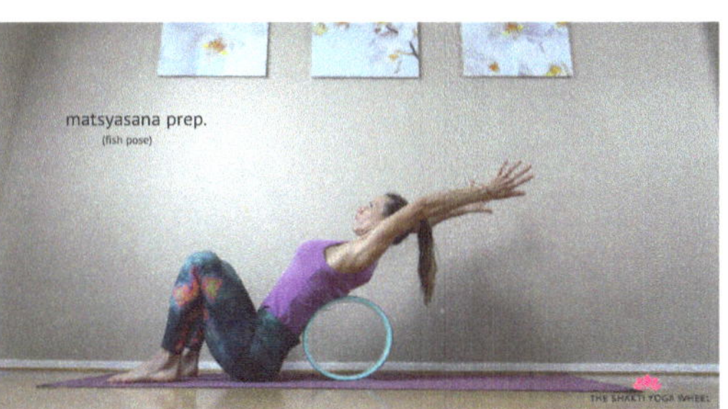

Matsayasana preparation - (fish pose)

Come to a seat with your knees bent and feet flat on the floor and parallel to each other. Place the wheel behind you along your spine. Draw the outer edges of your shoulder blades in toward the spine and lift the heart up, broadening the chest and collar bone. Exhale and draw your ribs down towards your hip points. Keeping your ribs drawing in and down, slowly lift your arms up over your head and curl back over your wheel. Spend several deep breaths here, rolling back and forth, melting into the wheel.

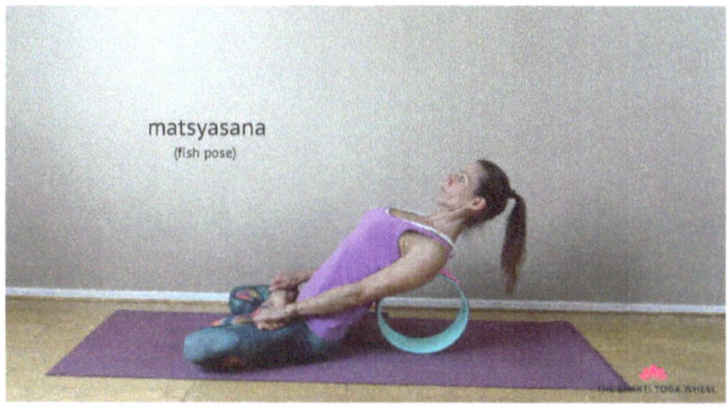

Matsayasana - (fish pose)

If padmasana, or lotus pose is in your practice, give this variation of fish pose a try. Begin seated with legs extended straight out in front of you. Bend your right knee and bring it in towards your chest, holding the leg in "baby cradle" for a few moments as you work the range of motion in the hip. Then, bring your right ankle to your left hip crease so the sole of your right foot faces the sky. Then, bend your left knee into "baby cradle" and rock it back and forth. Cross your left ankle over the top of your right shin. The sole of your left foot should also face upwards, and the top of your foot and ankle should rest on your hip crease. Draw your knees in and press your groins toward the floor. Sit up straight. If there is no pain in the ankle, knee or hip, stay here as you bring the wheel behind you and curl back over it. If you are uncomfortable here, release the legs from your lotus bind and go back to the previous pose.

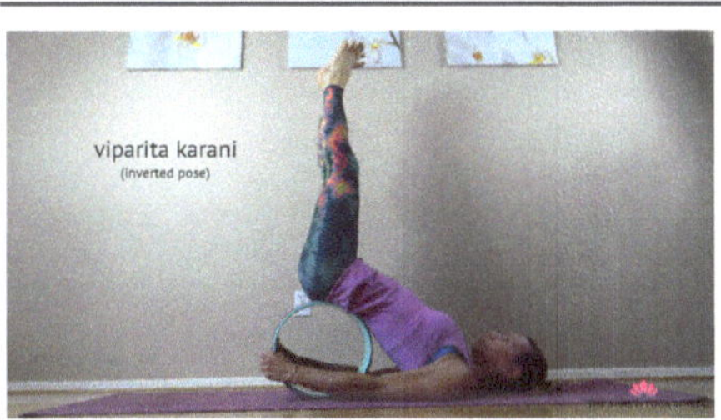

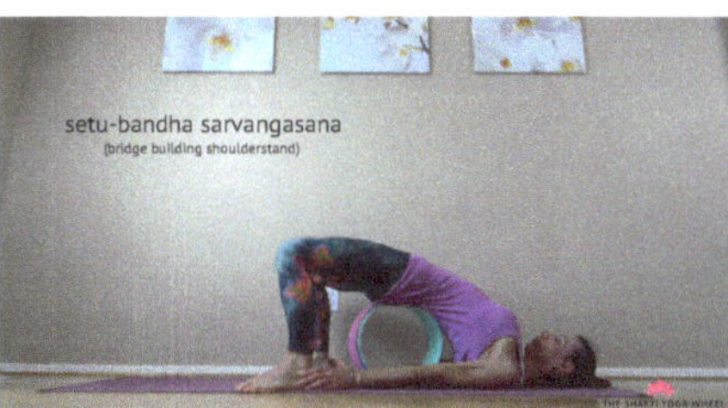

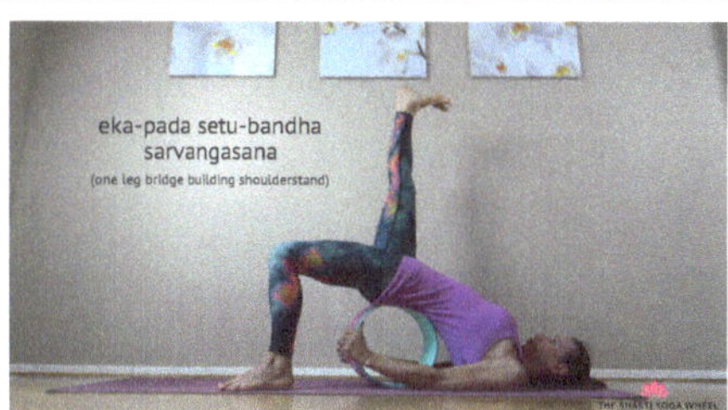

Viparita karani - (inverted pose)

Lie down on your mat, knees bent, and feet flat on the floor. Press into your feet and lift the hips up so you can slide the wheel under your sacrum. The wheel will sit nicely in the curve of your low back. Hug one knee in toward your chest and then the other, eventually extending both legs straight up to the sky. Reach your arms to your sides and grab hold of the wheel. Squeeze the shoulder blades in and lift your heart. Press the back of the skull into the mat to keep space between your chin and your chest.

Setu-bandha sarvangasana - (bridge building shoulderstand)

From viparita karani, bring the soles of the feet back to the mat and step them hip width distance apart and parallel. Squeeze the inner knees in and extend the arms to your sides, grabbing the wheel, or if you are able, grab your heels or outer ankles. Press into your heels. Allow the wheel to lift your heart and deepen your backbend while supporting your spine.

Eka-pada setu bandha sarvangasana - (one leg bridge building shoulderstand)

If you feel strong in the previous pose, try lifting one leg straight up to the sky. Press your triceps down to further lift the heart up. Continue pressing into the back of the skull.

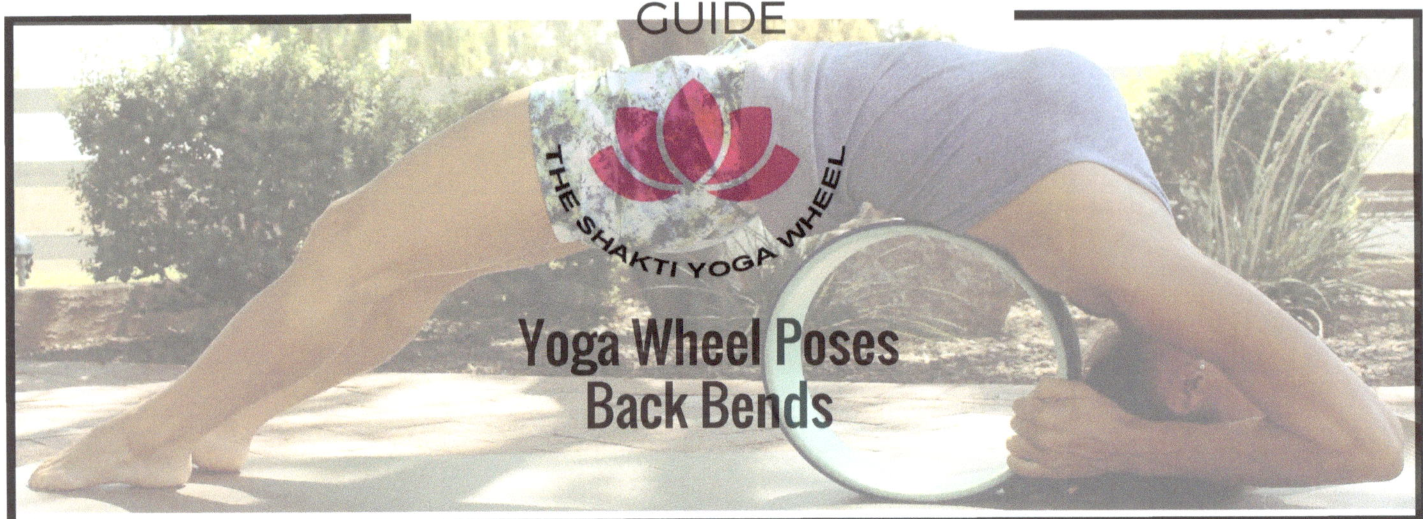

Yoga Wheel Poses
Back Bends

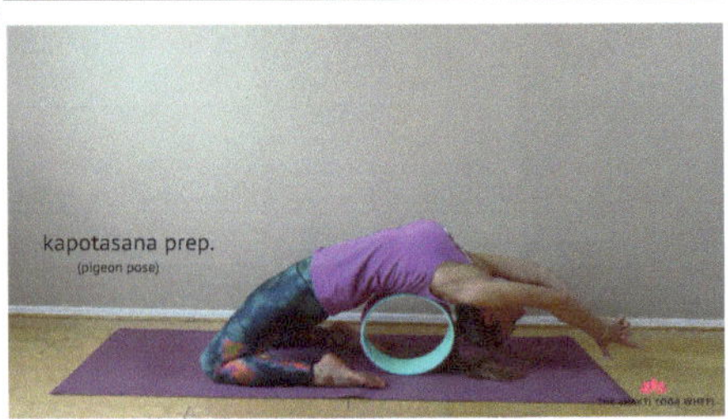

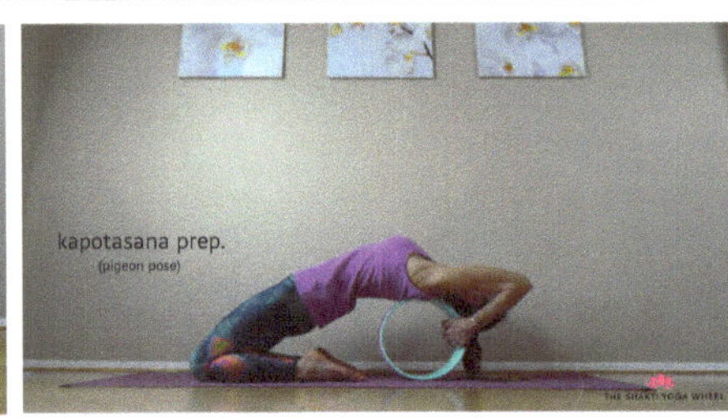

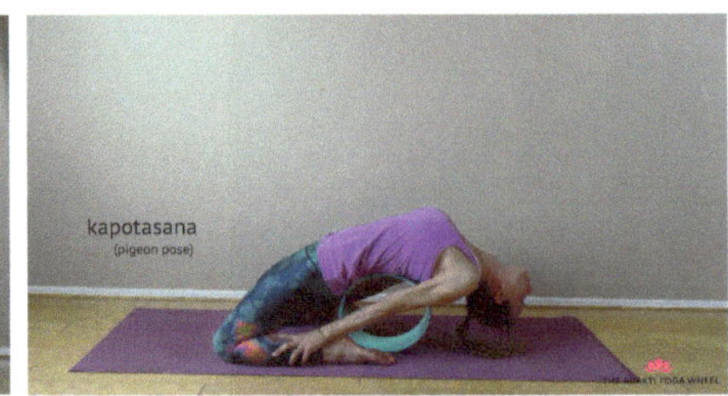

Kapotasana preparation - (pigeon pose prep.)
Begin kneeling on your mat, toes untucked so that the tops of the feet are on the mat. Narrow your hip points and narrow your ribs. Lean back so the upper back leans into your wheel. Reach the arms up and draw the arm bones deeper into the shoulder sockets. Continue to lift your arms overhead, keeping the ribs drawing down the armpits drawing in.

Kapotasana preparation - (pigeon pose prep.)
Now bend the elbows and grab the sides of the wheel. Squeeze the elbows in and plug the head of the arm bones deeper into the shoulder sockets, hollowing out the armpits. Press into your shins and the tops of your feet to lift your hips.

Kapotasana - (pigeon pose)
For the full pose, extend your arms to your sides and press into your heels or your calves. Lift your heart. You may want to roll the wheel from the upper back to the mid or low back. Always experiment with where the wheel is most supportive and comfortable for you. Keep the front of your body engaged as you curl back into this deep bend.

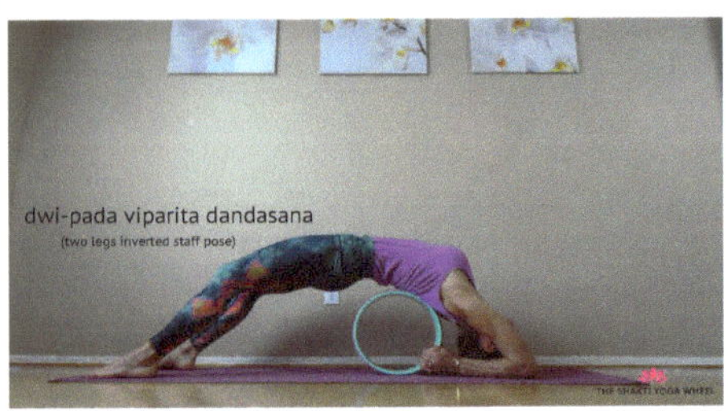

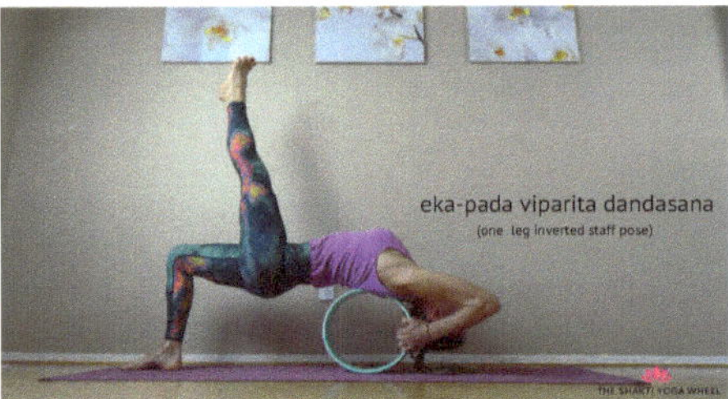

Dvi-pada viparita dandasana - (two legs inverted staff pose)
Begin in a seat, with your knees bent in front of you and your feet flat on the mat. Place the wheel behind you along your spine. Inhale the arms up and back, drawing the ribs down as you do so. Press into the feet to lift your hips up. Bend your elbows and grab the outer edges of the wheel. Lift your heels and press into the balls of the feet. Roll forward and back on your wheel, softening the chest and upper back. Roll forward until your elbows touch your mat. Exhale the ribs down and curl back deeper. Step the heels back down and root into the inner edges of your feet. This pose can be done with the legs bent or, you can walk your feet out, bringing the legs more towards straight. Plug the arm bones in.

Eka-pada viparita dandasana - (one leg inverted staff pose)
If you feel stable in the previous pose, draw to the midline and ground through one foot. Begin to feel lighter in the opposite foot. Bend the knee and hug the thigh into your chest. Extend the leg straight up to the sky. Breathe into the wheel and allow it to support you. Place the lifted leg down and lift the other leg.

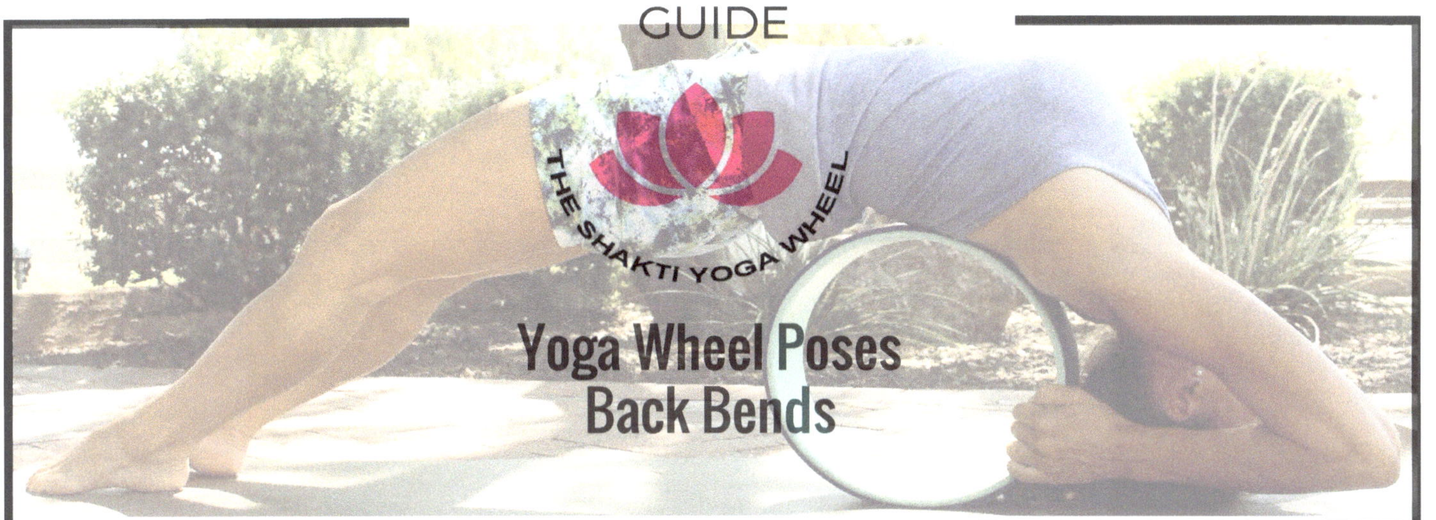

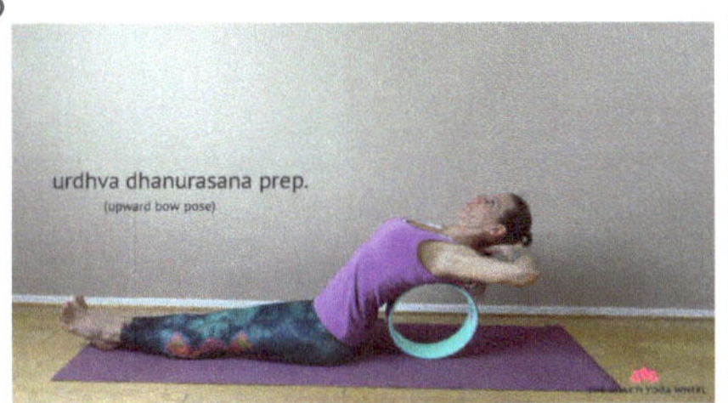

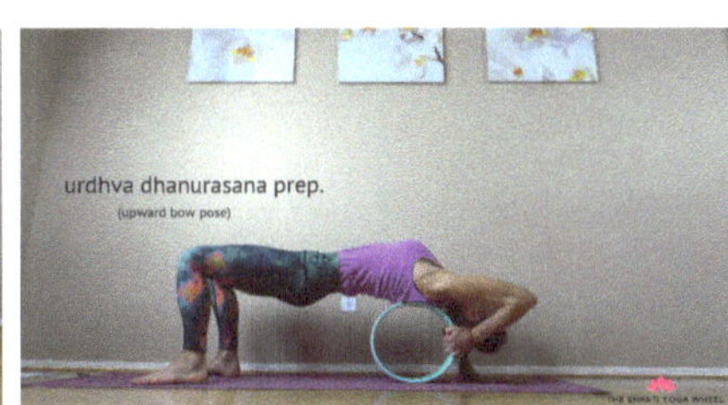

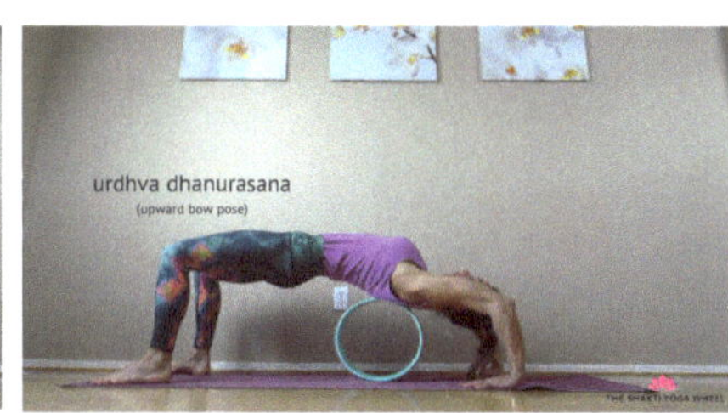

Urdvha dhanurasana preparation - (upward bow pose prep.)

Come to a seat with the legs extended straight out in front of you. Flex your feet. Whatever is touching the mat, press into those places. Be even on your sit bones and draw the thighs back. Exhale the ribs down and lift your arms up. Interlace the fingers behind the head. Stay here for several rounds of deep breaths, increasing the flexibility of the spine with every exhale.

Urdvha dhanurasana preparation - (upward bow pose prep.)

Next, bend the knees and press into the feet to lift the hips off the mat. Roll the wheel up and down along your spine, enjoying the massage the wheel gives your back muscles. Draw the ribs down and armpits in as you squeeze your elbows in toward each other. Grab the sides of the wheel. Hug the knees in and keep the inner thighs engaged. Drop the tops of your thighs down toward the mat, and then, press into your feet to lift your pelvis up again.

Urdvha dhanurasana - (upward bow pose)

Bring the palms to the mat, fingers pointing towards the shoulders. Squeeze your elbows in and hollow out the armpits. Press into the inner edges of your hands and press into your feet. Begin to straighten your arms as you lift your heart up and away from the wheel.

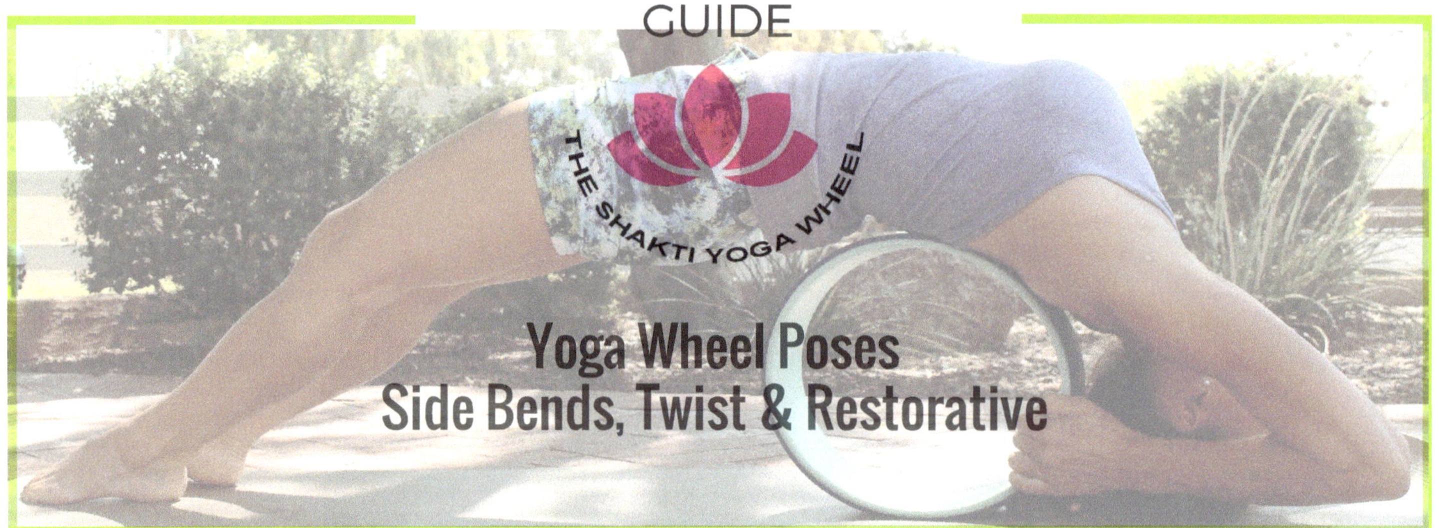

Yoga Wheel Poses
Side Bends, Twist & Restorative

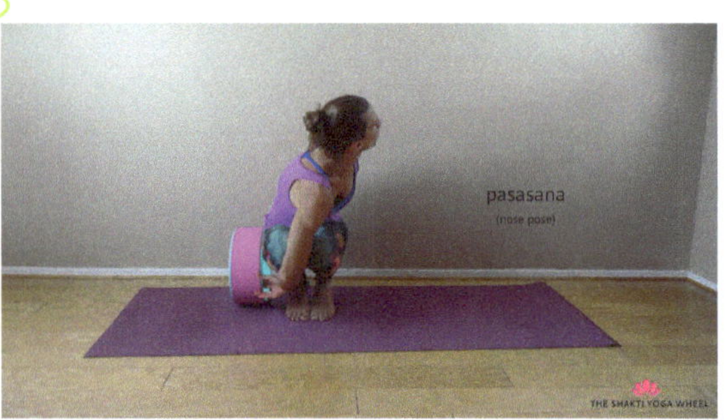

Pasasana - (noose pose)

In noose pose, the arms are wrapped around the squatting legs and the hands are clasped behind the back, forming a "noose." Begin standing in tadasana. Stand so that the inner edges of the feet are touching each other. Bend your knees into a full squat, keeping the inner knees touching. Keep the heels down, if possible. If you're not able to get the heels fully on the floor, squat with the heels raised on a folded blanket. Inhale and lengthen the spine.

Exhale and draw the navel to the spine, narrow the front ribs and twist toward one leg. If you practice this pose against a wall then you can use the wall for leverage to push and pull yourself deeper into the twist. Decrease the space between your ribs and the thighs. Reach your arms back and around you for the bind. If you cannot clasp your hands, grab the wheel instead. Breathe here for several deep breaths. Exhale to release. Twist to the other side.

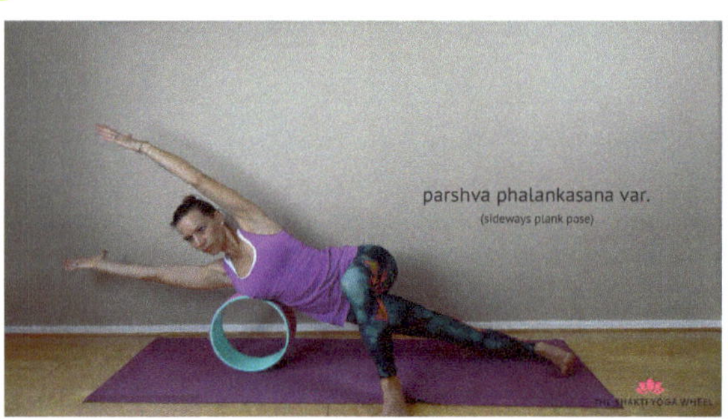

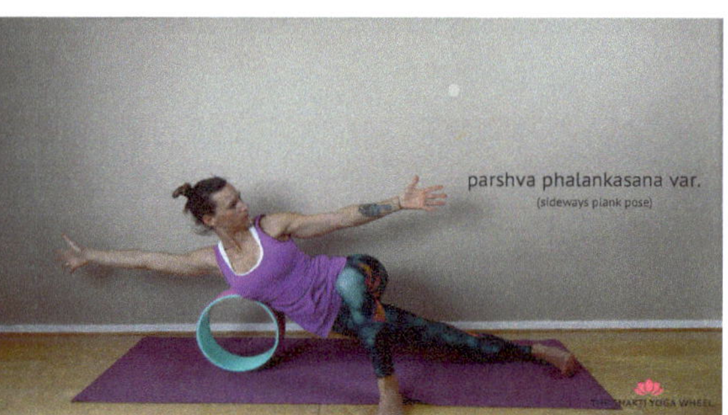

Parsva phalankasana- (sideways plank pose)

Begin seated on the outer strip of your right thigh with both hands on the mat in front of you. Bend your left leg and step the foot in front of the right straight leg. Place your wheel along the right side body, between the waistline and the armpit. Roll the wheel up and down until you find the most comfortable place to lean in to. Flex your back foot and press into the outer edge of the foot. Lift your hips up away from the mat. Lift both arms over head. Draw the ribs toward each other and down.

Parsva phalankasana variation - (sideways plank pose)

As a variation, you can sweep your top arm toward the back of the mat. Hold the pose for several breaths and switch sides.

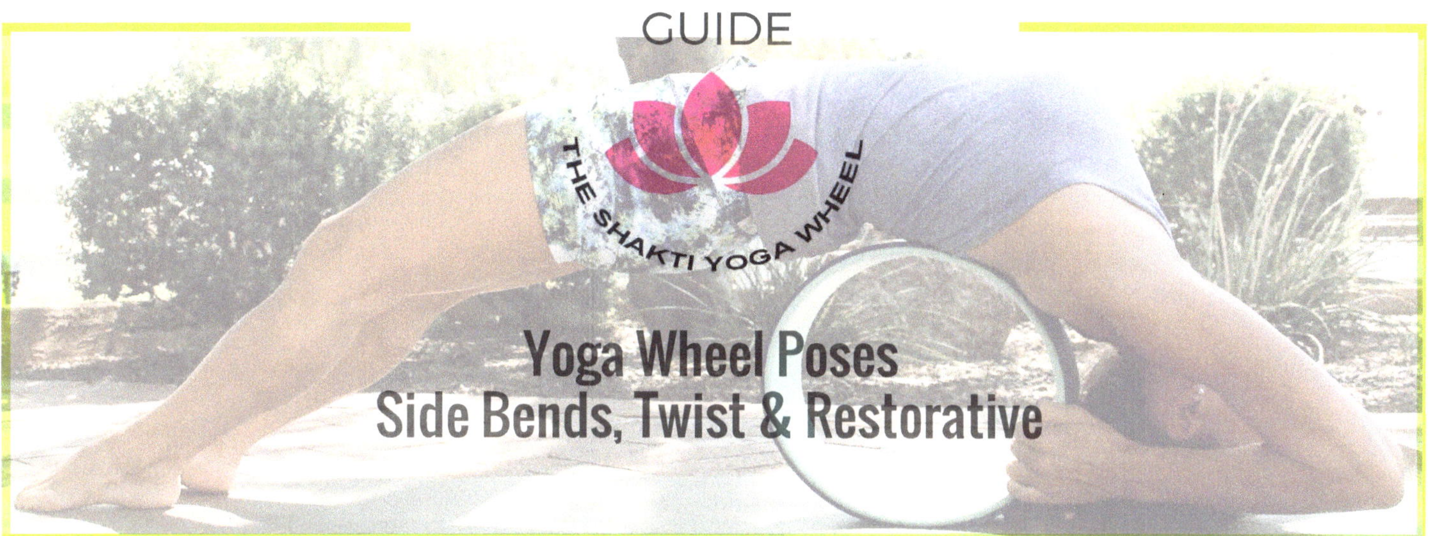

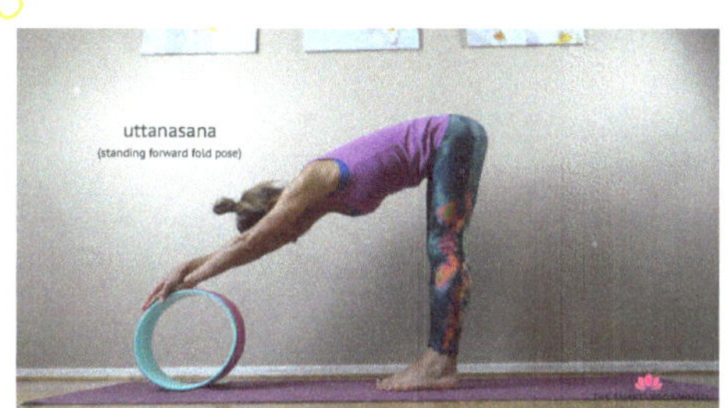

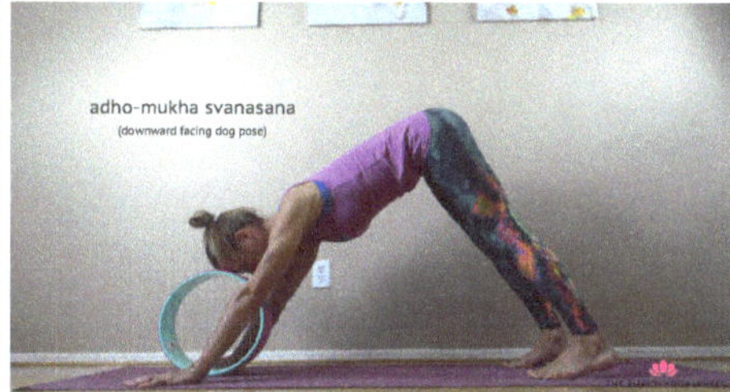

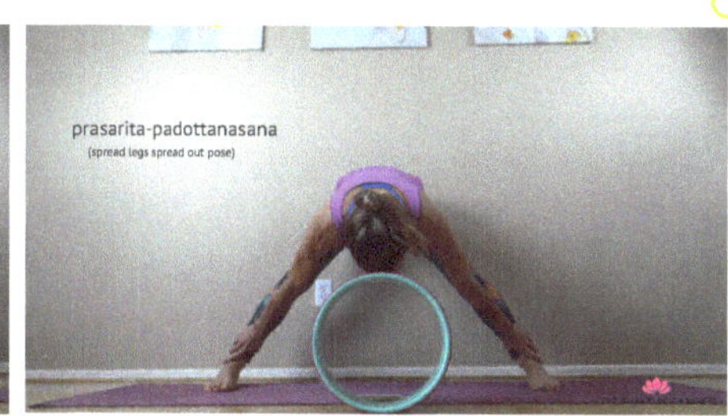

Uttanasana - (standing forward fold)
Come to standing with your feet hip width distance apart and parallel to one another. Lift and spread your toes to activate the muscles on the soles of the feet. Isometrically drag your heels back and lift up through the calf muscles. Press the tops of your shin bones forward and fold over your legs, grabbing your wheel with your hands. Place one hand on top of the other and slowly roll the wheel away from you. As you press the tops of your shin bones forward, take the tops of your thigh bones back. Lengthen your spine on an inhale. Exhale to narrow the front ribs. Stay here for several breaths. Then roll the wheel back in toward you and place the opposite hand on top. Roll the wheel forward again to stretch.

Adho mukha svanasana - (downward facing dog)
Come to hands and knees, with your hips directly over your knees and your shoulders directly over your wrists. Spread your fingers, and root down through the inner edge of your palms. Tuck your toes under and lift your knees away from the mat. Keep the knees slightly bent and the heels lifted away from the floor. Press into your hands and lengthen the heart towards the tops of the thighs. Then push the tops of your thighs back and draw your front ribs in. Roll your wheel to your head and rest the forehead on the wheel. If you come too much to the front of your forehead, the neck will over arch. If you come too much to the crown of your head, you will lose the natural curve in your cervical spine. Find a position that allows the head to be an extension of the spine. Lengthen through the top of your head and out through the base of your spine. Remain here for several deep breaths.

Prasarita padottanasana - (spread legs stretched out pose)
Stand wide on your mat, with the outer edges of your feet parallel to the short edges of your mat. Press into your feet and widen your heels apart. Lift the inner knee caps up and draw the inner thighs back and apart. Rest your forehead against your wheel just as you did in downward facing dog. Your hands can come to your outer shins, ankles or to the mat. Inhale to lengthen the spine.

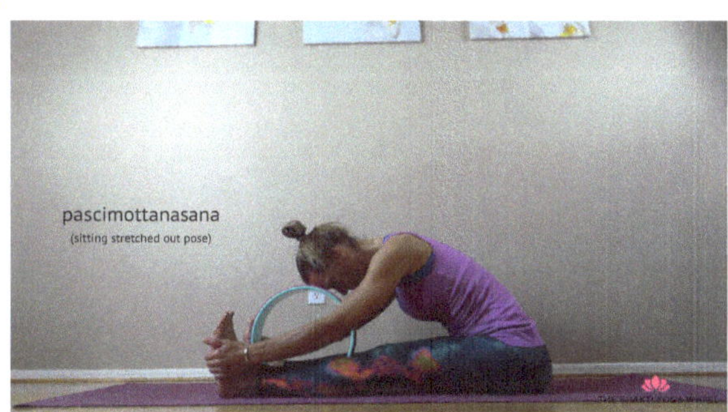

Pascimottanasana - (back stretched out pose)
Come to a seat with your legs extended out in front of you, sitting on the front of your sit bones. If your hamstrings are tight, sit up higher on a folded blanket. Place the wheel between your knees or shins. Sit up tall in the spine and bring your hands to the mat behind you. Press in to your finger tips and lift your heart up.

Hug the outer edges of your shoulder blades to midline. Exhale and hinge at the hips to slowly fold over your legs. Bring your forehead to the wheel. Avoid rounding your back. Close your eyes and soften into the stretch.

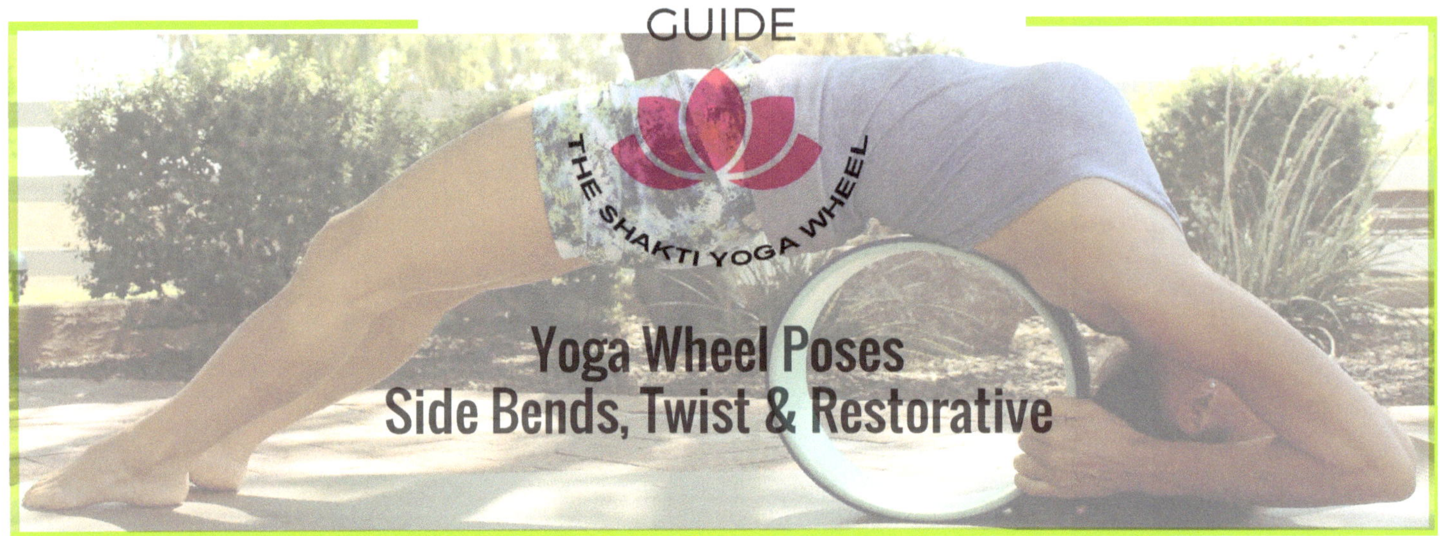

Yoga Wheel Poses
Side Bends, Twist & Restorative

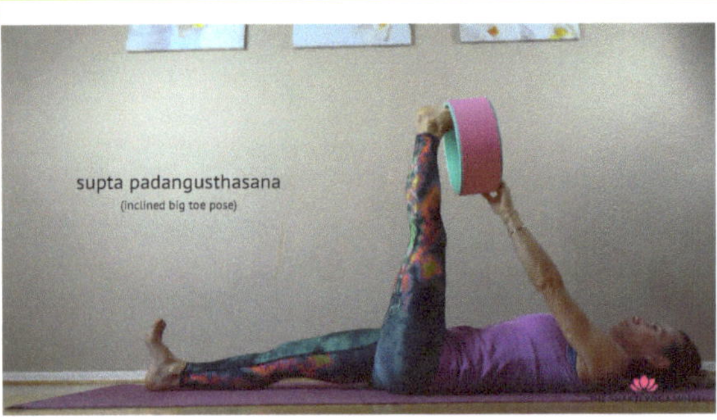

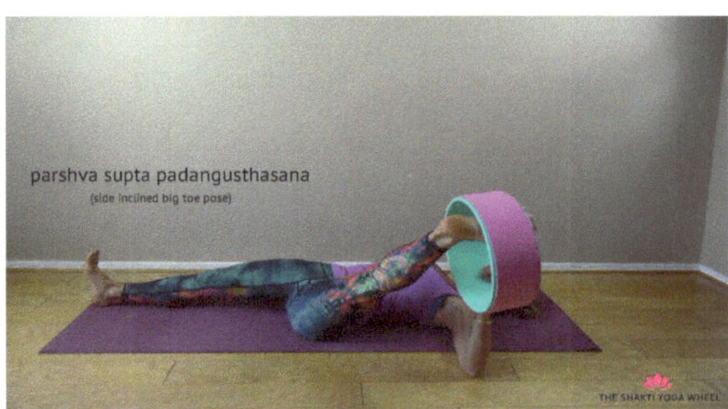

Supta padangusthasana - (reclined big toe pose)
Lie down flat on your back with both legs extended straight. Hug one knee into your chest and place the ball of the foot into the inner edge of the wheel. Hold on to the wheel with both hands and begin to straighten your bent leg straight up to the sky. For the first several breaths, bend and straighten this lifted leg to warm-up the hamstring. Then extend your leg straight, or as much towards straight as you can. Press the big toe mound into the wheel and press up through the inner heel. You can bend the bottom leg and place the sole of the foot flat on the mat to decrease the intensity of the stretch.

Parsva supta padangusthasana - (side reclined big toe pose)
After several breaths in the previous pose, hold the wheel in the hand that is the same side as the leg you are stretching. Bring your other hand to your side and rest it on the floor. Extend the lifted leg out to the side, bringing the wheel out with the foot. Just as in the previous pose, the bottom leg can be bent or straight. Rest your hand on top of the thigh to encourage the femur to remain grounded in the hip socket.

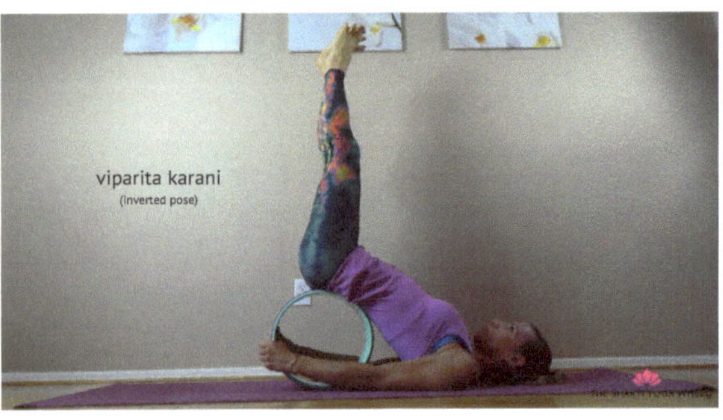

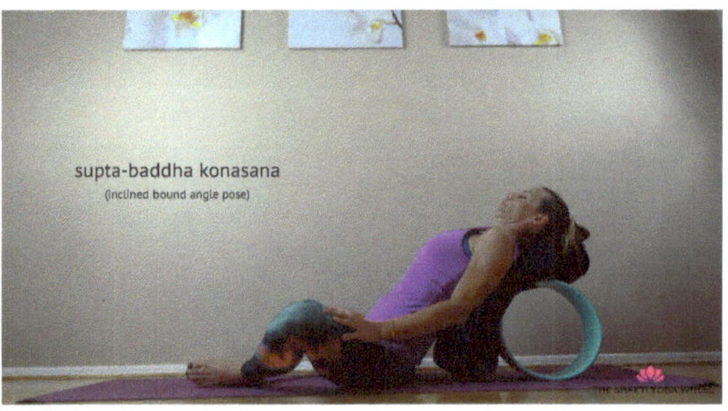

Viparita karani - (inverted pose)
Lie down on your mat, knees bent, and feet flat on the floor. Press into your feet and lift the hips up so you can slide the wheel under your sacrum. The wheel will sit nicely in the curve of your low back. Hug one knee in toward your chest and then the other, eventually extending both legs straight up to the sky. Reach your arms to your sides and grab hold of the wheel. Squeeze the shoulder blades in and lift your heart. Press the back of the skull into the mat to keep space between your chin and your chest.

Supta baddha konasana - (reclined bound angle pose)
Ah…we have saved the best for last! This blissful pose will leave you in love. In love with life. In love with your yoga wheel. And in love with this beautiful practice. For this pose you will need a bolster or several folded blankets. Begin seated in baddha konasana, with the soles of your feet together, and knees splayed out wide. Bring the wheel behind you and place the bolster between you and the wheel. Lie back into the wheel. If the wheel rolls away from you as you lean back in to it, rest the wheel against a wall. Release your arms to your sides and turn your palms up or, if more comfortable, rest them on your legs. Soften into the mat. Allow the wheel to support you. Close your eyes and stay here for as long as you would like.

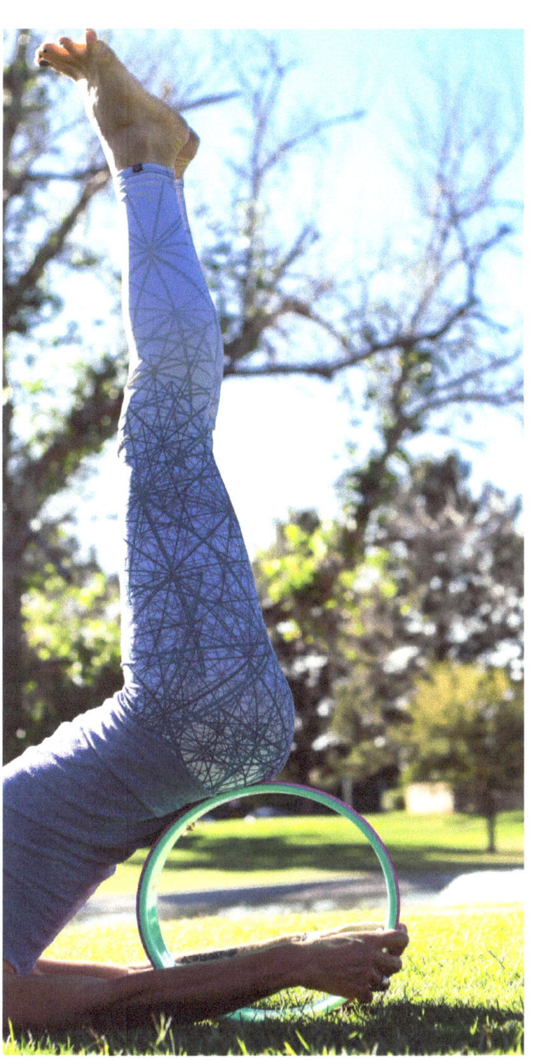

Thank You Note
& Authors

The Shakti Yoga Wheel™

The Shakti Yoga Wheel™ - 98 Posture Guide is dedicated to all the yogis who are sharing their words and actions of love and light into their communities. We are also grateful for many students, ambassadors, friends and family who have tested the Shakti Yoga Wheel™ itself and the guides and have given feedback and encouragement. The material and arrangement has slowly evolved and has imbued those who have been sincerely and deeply immersed in it with the conviction that The Shakti Yoga Wheel™ - 98 Posture Guide represents a completely new approach to find back into a natural and healthy posture.

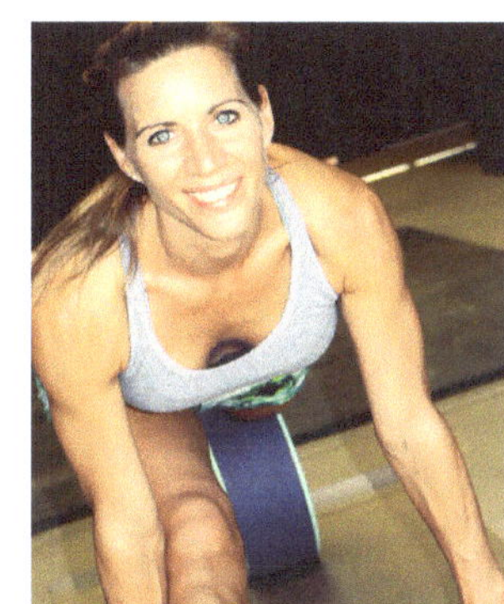

Jessyca Heinen-Collesei

is a E-RYT 500+, YACEP®, certified Jivamukti™, Ashtanga and Anusara Elements teacher, founder and director of Shakti Yoga & The Shakti Yoga Wheel™ .

Her work over the past few years has focused on supporting and mentoring the "next generation" of yoga students and teachers, through unwavering devotion to the spiritual teachings of yoga, clear cutting edge class content, and teaching playfulness on the Shakti Yoga Wheel to deepen and enhance the yoga practice. Jessyca lives in Arizona with her family and their two cats and horses. **www.shakti-flow-yoga.com**

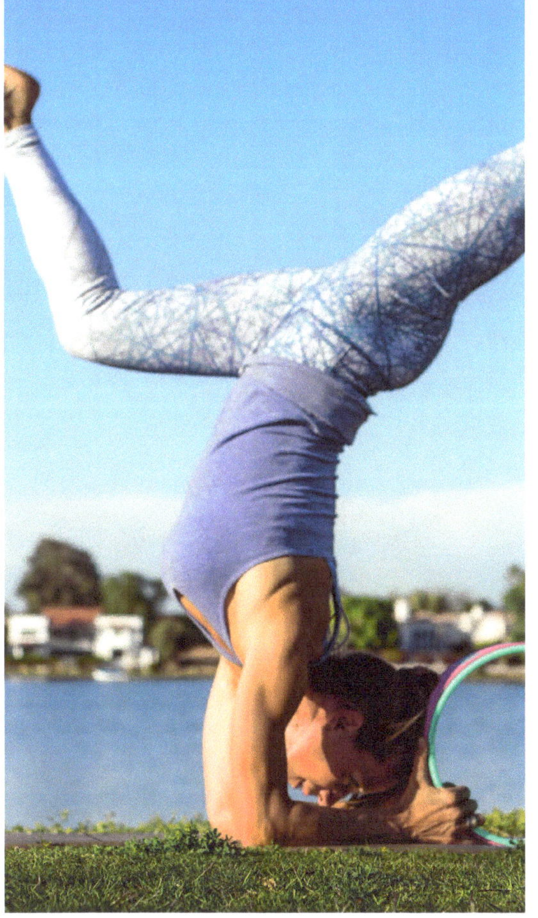

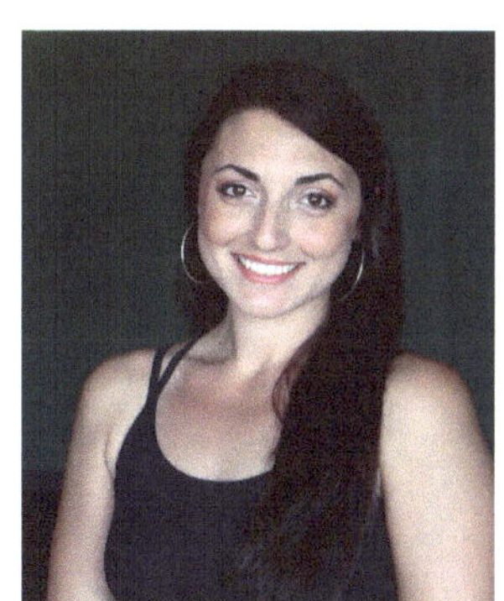

Elena Long

Teaches Anusara yoga, Vinyasa yoga, and kid's yoga in Fountain Hills and Scottsdale, Arizona. When she first saw a yoga wheel she knew she wanted to play around on it. Her favorite thing to do on the wheel is using it as a tool for passively working into backbends. It opens the chest and softens the upper back, prepping your body for deeper bending. And it feels so great! Her other favorite thing to do on the wheel is handstand press. Nothing will work your core and get you ready to press-up into a handstand quite like the yoga wheel.
www.elenalongyoga.com

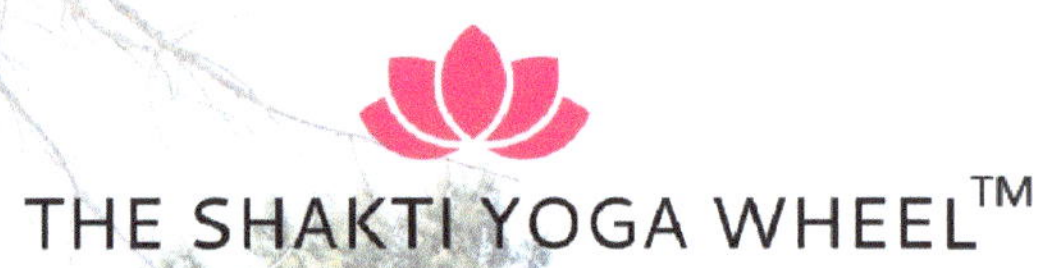

Intro

You need results? You want proof? Well, you found both, The Shakti Yoga Wheel™ is a light-weighted, easy to grip, portable resistance exerciser meant to improve your mobility, flexibility and strength; also for pregnancy, rehabilitation and strengthening shoulders, neck, spine and core. It has been proven in clinical study to reduce pain associated with reduced shoulder, lumbar and thoracic spine flexibility. The effect of self-myofascial and regaining strength is release on reduction of physical stress, speeding in healing of sport injuries, increased range of motion, muscle recovery, and performance. The effect of self-myofascial release is the reduction of physical stress. The Shakti Yoga Wheel™ is a true breakthrough and it's costs a lot less than other much less effective options. Because we do research and make products to professional standards. The Shakti Yoga Wheel™ is the #1 exercise tool to open up the shoulders, neck and back among yoga professionals and athletes.

Important Safety Information

 This is the safety alert symbol. It is used to alert you to important safety information. To avoid accidents and personal injuries, read and obey all safety messages that follow this symbol.

Before each use of the Shakti Yoga Wheel™, follow these instructions:

- Consult your physician before starting any exercise program. Children, pregnant moms and persons with medical conditions should not use this product unless first approved by a physician.
- This Product Contains ABS (acrylonitrile), TPE and Dry Natural Rubber. Some persons may be allergic. Stop using if you notice any reaction.
- The exercise tips shown in this brochure are guidelines. They do not replace any instructions or directions provided by a doctor or therapist.
- Do not load more weight then recommended.
- Inspect the product for any damage before each use. Discard and replace a damaged product.
- This product is not a toy. Keep out of reach for children or pets.

When using the Shakti Yoga Wheel™, always follow these instructions:

- If you have any dizziness, trouble breathing, increasing pain or begin to feel sick with the exercise, stop and contact your healthcare provider immediately.
- Children should only use if prescribed by a doctor, and only with adult supervision.

Caring for the Shakti Yoga Wheel™:

- Inspect after each use. Discard and replace the product if damaged.
- To Clean: Use a mild soap and warm water to clean. Then pat dry.
- Store it in a cool, dry place, out of direct sunlight and extreme temperatures.

Product offering

Max weight: 397 lbs
Recommended sizes: 4-6 feet tall
Weight/Width/Diameter: 3.5 lbs / 5.1 inch/ 12.5 inch

Research Proven Exercises

Mobility, flexibility and strengthening exercises are designed to improve the mobility, flexibility, strength and endurance of muscles that either may not functioning properly because of an injury or condition, or that may have simply weakened over time. Mobility, flexibility or strengthening exercises should not be painful or extremely difficult. Generally, theses exercises should be performed at a light to moderate intensity level (2 to 5 on a scale of 10) – ideally working 2-3 sets of 2-5 repetitions, 3 times per week.